lazy loser

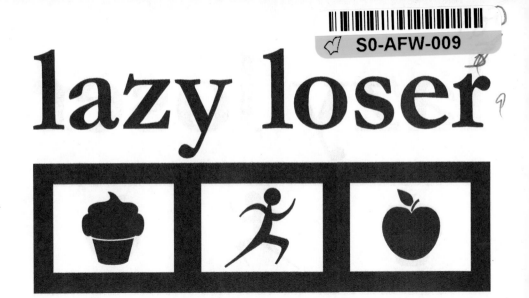

To Dorothy

Happy Losing

M

lazy loser

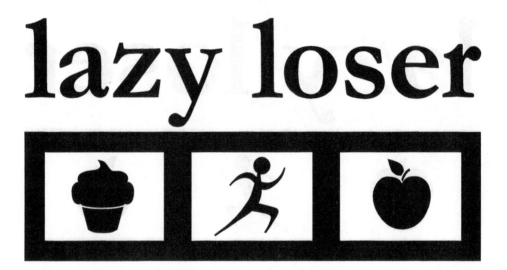

First Published 2013 by Lazy Runner Pty Ltd, PO Box 1308, Noosa Heads, Queensland 4567, Australia

Disclaimer

Whilst every effort has been made to ensure the content of the Lazy Loser book is accurate and sound as possible. Neither the author nor the publishers can accept responsibility for any injuries, illness or health problems sustained as a result of following the information, training programs or eating and drinking suggestions contained in this Lazy Loser book.

The author strongly recommends that any person starting out on a new eating plan or fitness activity, consult a health care professional, to rule out any underlying problems or medical conditions that could be affected by the new activity or eating plan.

All information on nutrition and diet has been researched by the author and taken from her life experiences of her own lifestyle and nutritional needs, and should be used as a general guideline only as everyone's nutritional and health needs are different. The Author is not a qualified dietician or nutritionist.

The author and publishers have made every effort to contact copyright holders for the material used in this book. Any person or organisation that has been overlooked should contact the publisher.

Author: Bean, Marie, author.
Title: Lazy loser / Marie Bean.
ISBN: 9780987386526 (paperback)
Series: Bean, Marie, Lazy runner ; 2
Subjects: Weight loss.
Health.
Physical fitness.
Dewey Number: 613.25

ISBN 978-0-9873865-2-6
Design by Steve Williams, Red Inc.
Illustrations by Thomas Barnett
Printed by Griffin Press

To buy copies of this book please contact

www.lazyrunner.com

This book is dedicated to an amazing lady –
My Wonderful Mother
Margaret Lyons

Contents

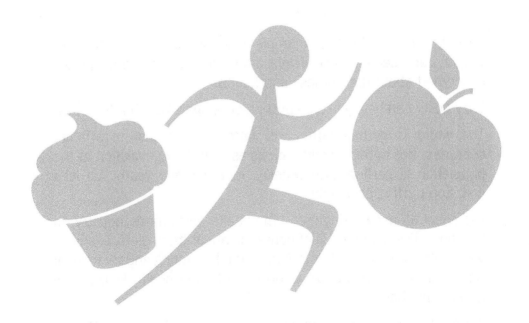

Introduction

I'm not a dietician or nutritionist, which is okay, as this book is not about diet or nutrition.

I'm not a food scientist, which is okay, as this book is not about the science of food.

I'm not a chef or food economist, which is okay, as this isn't a healthy cookbook (plus, I'm the world's worst cook).

I'm not a Skinny Bitch (well, not the first bit anyway!), which is okay, as this book is not about how to be one.

I'm not a health nut, which is okay, as this book is not about wheatgrass shots and tofu (and I like chocolate too much).

I'm not a kick-butt fitness fanatic, which is okay, as this book isn't about inflicting pain in an effort to get fit.

You're probably wondering how I could write a book about staying healthy, eating well, and losing weight if I'm not an expert in any of the above fields. If it helps, I do know lots about food — eating it, that is!

This is not a weight-loss book; you won't lose weight by reading it (in my defence, though, you won't lose weight by reading any book — even the diet ones).

Lazy Loser is a book for people who are unhappy with their weight, can't seem to lose weight after a lifetime of trying, and are concerned about their fitness and health.

Lazy Loser can help you stop putting on weight. Hey, that's a start!

The world is getting fatter and fatter — not just in affluent countries, but in third-world nations as well. A huge section of the population is getting fatter weekly, monthly, and yearly. So let's just stop putting on weight.

I've spent all my working life in the health-and-fitness industry. In that time, I've heard loads of nonsense about food, diets, exercise, and health. I've decided to toss my hat into the ring and try to instil some sanity into this crazy world of diets and health kicks. Lazy Loser is my hat.

I'm not fat, but I'm not thin either. Over the past 17 years (a year after the birth of my fourth child), I've remained the same weight, give or take a few kilos. My ideal weight for my height is 68 kg, and I hover between 65 and 67 kg. I say hover, but I really don't know as I only weigh myself a few times a year, but each time I get on a scale I'm usually within that range.

And before you ask, no, I'm not naturally thin. I was a fat child and teenager. I've dieted and failed many times in the past; and, I'm not an organic, free-range vegan. I love meat, chocolate, and a tipple (yes, in that order, and quite often).

How have I done it then?

Years ago, I discovered a formula that works for me. I like food — lots of it, and often not the lowest-calorie varieties. That's the easy bit . . . but how do I indulge without getting fat?

I enjoy outdoors activities. A long time ago, I taught myself how to run and I don't mind doing that, especially if it means I don't have to give up my favourite foods.

That's it, really! So how do I get a book out of a two-sentence formula?

It's all about sticking to the formula for life — and life can be tricky. Things change, our lives get busy and chaotic, new food choices and temptations are in our faces daily, and confusion over what's good for us and what's not is rife in our society.

Over the years, my formula has been tweaked. If I'm training for a big race (I started running ultra-marathons last year, in my 50s), I can eat more; that's the good part. However, I also have to choose healthy foods and give up some of my favourite things, like alcohol, as I need lots of energy to get me through my running events.

Then there are the times when I go home for Christmas. I can easily enter my mother's house on Boxing Day and waddle out New Year's Day, with a bit of extra baggage to take home (and I'm not talking about the checked kind). This situation leads to a week or two of cutting back on rich foods and running farther or more often.

I'm not sure how much weight I gained or lost on these occasions, but I did know that the formula was a bit askew and had to be put back in order. How did I know after my mother's Christmas spread? I felt sluggish and lacking in energy, my clothes were a bit tight; running wasn't as easy as it usually is for me, etc. Once I was back to my normal formula, all was well again — no deprivation or hard work — and within a couple weeks, I was feeling good with the extra baggage gone.

I know I make it sound simple, but that's because it is, once you get to the place I'm at: Knowing what works for you and sticking to it for life. Lazy Loser is about finding the right formula for you.

It starts with you stopping putting on weight; that's number one. You don't wake up one morning 10 kg overweight; it happens over months or years, and there's something in your eating, drinking, and exercise (or lack of) habits that's causing that slow weight gain.

When you've halted the gaining, it's time to get to the weight you want to be. No, it's not the sizes you see in magazines: The under-15s on the beach in their bikinis or the boys with six packs; it's the size that is right for you. Often, it's a size you've been before in your adult life. This is the size and shape you need to work on — not the stick insect, media portrayal body that you, me and 90% of the population will never be.

Lazy Loser is not a work of fiction, and you'll be reminded of that constantly as you read on; it's best to deal with facts and reality if you want this to work.

When you start on your Lazy Loser plan, your next question will be, "How long will it take?"

Let me ask you a question: How long have you got?

I'm hoping you have a lifetime, as that's how long it'll take: A lifetime of eating and drinking, good health, and no dieting. Surely that sounds like something you could live with forever.

Once you work out how to stop putting on weight, you'll probably already have an idea of what your Lazy Loser plan is. Then it's a matter of tweaking this formula into a weight loss for you. One little tweak could amount to no loss in a week, but it may mean half a kilo a month, which will turn into 6 kg (13 lb) a year — not bad for not even trying.

What's a tweak? It's something minor you're doing that could be the reason you're putting on weight.

Giving up your fruit juice with breakfast each morning = 5 kg (11 lb) of weight loss a year.

Reducing your two sugars back to one in three cups of tea or coffee a day = 3 kg (6.5 lb) a year.

Adding one extra hour of exercise a week and doing nothing else = 3 to 4 kg (6–8 lb) a year, depending on the activity.

You may think only 3 kg a year is not much reward, but look at what you're doing to get it: Hardly anything. No sacrifice, deprivation, or torture — just leading your normal life. And remember: The figures are on these little things; you could up the ante and tweak two things in your life to lose double the kilos over the year.

Look back and work out how long it took you to get fat. It could have been five to 10 years, so you have plenty of time to work on going in the other direction.

I wrote "Lazy Loser" to dispel some crazy myths and perceptions when it comes to food and fitness. Some of these are:

• Bad food. No food is bad, evil, or mean. Food is wonderful and delicious, and all can make you fat if you overindulge; some food makes you fatter more quickly than others.

• Super foods. No food has superpowers to make you thinner, fitter, or drop weight faster. Some foods are healthy and some not so healthy, but it all goes in one end and out the other.

• Energy in (food and drink) versus energy out (daily movement and exercise) is still the only formula you need to look at for weight gain and loss. It's been around for years and it's not going to change in our lifetimes; accept this fact and work with it.

• You don't have to overhaul your life (or your fridge and pantry) to lose weight and get healthy. It's likely that only 20–30% of what you're doing is causing you to gain weight. These are the areas that need to be focused on.

• Diets don't work and never will, so stop trying them.

• The bottom line is that we eat too much, too often — these things that can be easily tweaked.

• There are many choices and temptations in the 21st century — lots more than in our parents' and grandparents' day. However, the food they cooked and ate is still out there. Sometimes it's hard to find, so don't bother looking too much in the supermarket aisles; stick to the perimeter of the store, or get to the green grocer or farmers' market.

• Fat genes, hormones, fat parents who force-fed us rubbish, emotional eating, etc.: The excuse list is never-ending. Writing down your fat excuse is not going to help; you still have to go through the same process as everyone else if you want to lose weight.

• If reading labels, counting calories, and obsessing about the nutritional values of packaged foods is driving you crazy and causing confusion, stop doing those things. There are other ways to sort out the best method for you to stay in control of what you eat and how you move.

Lazy Bottom Line

I haven't met you and I know nothing of your struggles, or the ups and downs you've had in the past with eating, diets, and weight-loss failures. However, I'm writing this book for you. I've met many people over the years who've struggled with their weight, and I've heard all their horror diet histories, so I do know lots of people like you.

I have five simple goals that I hope you achieve from reading "Lazy Loser":

1. You see yourself in sections of this book: You can relate to some of the things I talk about, and recognise that you've fallen into the bad habits and food traps I write about.

2. You find three things in this book you know you can incorporate into your life right now without causing major overhauls or drama, or spending buckets of money.

3. You gain confidence to take charge of the food you eat, beverages you drink, and how you incorporate fitness in your life without feeling pressured, stressed, or guilty. You end up doing what suits your lifestyle, and maybe even enjoy it as well.

4. You determine your own special formula to stop gaining weight, start losing weight, and get on the road to a long, healthy, happy, normal life to become the ultimate Lazy Loser.

5. You have a chuckle and see the lighter side of this crazy, fat world we live in.

"Lazy Loser" is about you and your formula. Throughout the book, you'll read bits about me and my experiences; however, this is not about changing you into me. You don't have to take up running or eat the way I do. The best thing is to see how to alter your food and exercise choices to suit your preferences, so you get a system that works for you like mine does for me.

As you're reading "Lazy Loser", you may find the advice and suggestions basic, simplistic, and boringly normal, but that's a big thumbs-up for me — it means you understand my Lazy ideas and I've got my message across. Eating, drinking, and moving are the background scene of your life.

I wanted to put those things back in their place, so the focus can be on the main event: Living life to the fullest and having fun!

Enjoy – and happy Lazy Losing!

Marie

Chapter 1 – My Big Fat Rant

I will get my fat rant out in the open early-then we can all move on!

Latest figures show Australia as one of the fattest nations in the world, with over 4 million Aussies overweight or obese (that is 60% of the population). Of that number, 123,000 will die within the next 20 years purely from complications related to their obesity. The most likely diseases are heart disease, stroke, and diabetes.

Obesity is the leading preventable cause of premature death in the world, and has just passed smoking as the most preventable cause of death in Australia. Diseases caused by obesity are now at over 8%, and smoking is slowly decreasing, sitting at 6.8%. It's estimated that these figures are trending worldwide.

Not only are we fatter than we've ever been — we continue to get heavier. By 2020, an estimated 80% of Australians will be overweight or obese. We are not at our peak and yet we're doing very little to stem the fat tide or reverse it.

One of the reasons smoking and the diseases it causes have decreased is because we stopped tolerating the habit in society. The anti-smoking campaign has worked very well. It took time, money and lots of legal wrangling, but the results speak for themselves.

However, now that smoking looks to be taking a back seat to obesity in terms of health risk and disease, the same amount of effort and campaigning is not being directed at this new risk that is affecting far more people.

Society and health officials treat smokers very differently from the obese. Smokers claim they've been ostracised, abused, and outcast from society for their bad habit; however, society accepts and even encourages our overeating and unhealthy food culture. Both health risk groups knowingly put things into their mouths that may eventually kill them.

If you go to a doctor and he/she learns you're a smoker, a stern lecture would ensue; in a lot of cases you are refused treatment and surgery in hospital unless you've butted out, which is rightly enforced.

Compare the way Australia deals with both these major health hazards:

Smoking and Cigarettes	Unhealthy Foods and Drinks
Cost: Expensive, and going up all the time. There are never sales or discounts on cigarettes.	Cost: Cheap (buy two chocolate bars for the price of one, upsize your meal deals for more fat and sugar). Fizzy drinks are cheaper than bottled water, and potato chips are cheaper than fruit.
Size: Can only buy one packet at a time (cartons no longer sold).	Size: Supersize me, buy as much as you want; the more you buy, the cheaper it is.
Availability: Cigarettes are out of sight and (hopefully) out of mind; they are locked away in cupboards, and only come out if you ask for them.	Availability: In your face. Don't worry if you missed picking up your lolly fix in the supermarket aisles — it will be waiting for you at the checkouts.
Social: You can smoke only in designated areas, and mostly outdoors.	Social: Eat and drink anytime, anywhere: At the office, on the street, in your car, etc.

Labelling: Graphic, ugly images on all packs and brand names have been removed.	Labelling: Gorgeous, slim models eating and drinking, and seeming not to be gaining any weight.
Advertising: Total ban on cigarette advertising.	Advertising: Everywhere: Billboards, TV (even during kids' programs), magazines, newspapers, and sporting events.
Sponsorship deals: Tobacco brands cannot sponsor any company or sporting group.	Sponsorship deals: Fast-food and soft-drink companies sponsor major events, even sporting events and clubs.
Government campaigns: Highly successful quit campaign; from 1980 to 2013, smoking in Australian adults has dropped from 35% to 16%.	Government campaigns: Every now and then we see a government-sponsored campaign for exercising 30 minutes a day or eating the recommended five vegetable/ two fruit servings a day. But we never see an ad or billboard telling us to quit junk food or soft drinks, or showing us the effect they have on our health.
Tax: A packet of cigarettes in Australia is taxed more than 53%.	Tax: Apart from GST, no other taxes as yet. There is talk of a 20% fat tax on fast food and soft drinks, but it hasn't been put into action yet.
Deaths: 15,531 deaths are attributed annually to effects of smoking and the number is falling.	Deaths: 9,500 deaths are attributed annually to the effects of obesity, and the number is rising.
Cost to society and government: $31 billion and falling.	Cost to society and governments: Estimated $37.7 billion and rising.

If the statistics are correct, more than 80% of us will be overweight or obese by 2020. Shouldn't we be ramping up our concern about this? There is a lot of talk about the number of us getting fatter; discussions on how bad the food industry is; and many facts about the diseases that will arise as a result, but very little action being taken to manage this obesity crisis. The latest craze is trying to find the fat gene and then inventing a drug to deal with it. But is that the real answer?

What about some regulations on the big food and drink companies who keep churning out empty-calorie, high-sugar, high-fat foods at tiny prices and never once mentioning the health risks that could be associated with their products — the same thing we did with cigarettes? At least that would be a start.

I am not a fan of taxing unhealthy food, but what about making healthy food more accessible and as cheap as the unhealthy variety? Then money won't be an issue when it comes to making good food choices.

Many people, think it's okay to overeat, make poor food choices, be inactive and, as a result, be fat. If society's tolerance was lower (as it is with smoking), would overweight or obese people be more inclined to do something about their weight? Right now, the mindset is, "When we grow out of our clothes, go to the plus-sized department." I've even heard that airlines are going to make bigger seats due to the increase in the population's weight. Is that the answer — making everything bigger?

We've become desensitised to our own fat and the fat around us, and this will worsen the larger we all get. As society gets bigger, soon overweight people will look thinner, and compare themselves to the morbidly obese, saying, "Oh well, at least I'm not as big as that guy."

Eat Breakfast and Live Longer! A survey of 26,902 US male health professionals over 16 years to monitor health- during that time 1,572 of the participants had some form of cardiac event. The survey found that the men who didn't eat breakfast had a 27% higher risk of heart attack or death from a coronary disease than the male breakfast eaters.

Ultimately, as adults, we are all in charge of our own health and food choices, so if we're fat, we have only one person to blame. However, as a society, there is a lot more that could be done to help us make the healthier, right choices — especially for children and teenagers, who are very susceptible to making poor food choices.

Some ideas are:

• Regulating the amount of sugar and salt added to processed foods and drinks.

• Stopping the dominance of fast/unhealthy food advertising, especially at sporting events or during children's TV viewing times.

• Regulating or replacing trans-fat content in processed and fast foods.

• Reducing the price of fruit and vegetables so they are on par with the cheaper packaged food prices.

• Making food labelling less complicated.

• Give all foods a health rating, making it big and bold, and stick it on the front (like with cigarette package warnings).

• Introducing education programs in schools and for new parents on how to eat well, exercise, and stay healthy.

Lazy Tale

Let me tell you about my hometown doctor. He was your old-school, grumpy variety family GP. Visits to him usually lasted less than 15 minutes with as little verbal communication as possible, and you were never in the room for more than two minutes before he had you up on the examination table "having a poke around" (his medical terminology, not mine).

He only ever told you as much as he thought you should know; however, there was something comforting about the way he took charge. If he told you that you were going to be all right, you were — and if you were going to die, he would tell you that too.

When I was six months pregnant with my second child, Jonathon, 26 years ago, I felt really bad. I was still working as a nurse, had three months until my due date, and felt like I was ready to drop. I had a bad back, puffy ankles, severe indigestion; I was always tired and had no energy. It was not good.

At my six-month check-up, I sat in the waiting room with a list of my symptoms. I was convinced that Doc would tell me to leave work, rest for the next three months, be waited on hand and foot, and eat as much comfort food as possible (maybe the last two would be pushing it a tad!).

I lumbered into the Doc's surgery. He looked at the list and told me to get up on the examination table (you know, for the "poke-around").

When he finished, I said, "Give it to me straight, Doc — what is wrong with me?"

His diagnosis was two words:

"You're fat."

I wouldn't have been more shocked if he slapped me with his stethoscope. "I'm having a baby!" I cried in indignation.

He then proceeded to pinch mounds of my flesh, starting with one on my back. "Is this baby?" he asked. Then he moved on to my legs. "Is this baby?"

"No," I whimpered.

"Just because you're having a baby doesn't give you a license to eat and drink for two," he said. "You've gained more than enough weight for not just one, but two pregnancies. You're not going to gain one more kilo for the rest of this pregnancy."

"What? My baby will starve!"

"He won't starve, he is big and healthy, and you will get fatter and more unwell if you keep going like this"

He told me all my symptoms were coming from my obesity, and that they would escalate if I didn't do something about it.

He referred me to a dietician to get a healthy pregnancy eating plan and more information on eating and exercising during pregnancy.

I was shocked, embarrassed, and angry. But after I calmed down, I thought, *Come on, at least your baby is okay, and he wouldn't say those things to you if they're wrong, or if he didn't care.*

However, I still wasn't convinced that I wasn't seriously ill, but I thought, *I'll show you. I'll do everything you say, and prove that it's not fat causing all my problems!*

I followed the advice the dietician gave me. I started eating right, walking daily, and I continued to work. I didn't put on any more weight throughout the pregnancy, and guess what? All my nasty symptoms left. I continued to work for another two months, went full term, had a huge, healthy baby boy, and got back to my pre-pregnancy weight within a couple of months.

I know being told you're fat is a hard, bitter, and embarrassing pill to swallow. But the most important thing is to stop associating the fat word with other terms like horrible, grotesque, or ugly. Being overweight or obese is a harmful condition, and needs to be addressed so you can live a long, healthy, and disease-free life.

This book is my small attempt to turn the tide on obesity. If the powers that be are going to keep telling us that being fat is a dangerous condition and yet not be prepared to take on and solve some of the issues aggravating it, so be it. Let's sort out our own backyards and in turn, improve our own health.

Lazy Bottom Line

- As a society we're getting fatter. 60% of the population is overweight or obese, and that is forecast to hit 80% by 2020.

- Being overweight or obese can be a major contributing cause to most of the killer diseases of the western world: Heart disease, cancer, diabetes, and stroke.

- Little is being done by food manufacturers, health officials, or governments to turn the tide and start effective campaigns to decrease weight gain and improve our general health.

- The anti-smoking campaigns have been very successful; maybe health and government officials could adapt some of that hard sell to help solve the obesity crisis.

- Children are getting fatter and unhealthier, and may not live as long as their parents. That is very sad and scary, and should be of great concern to all of us.

- We need to take charge of our own health (and our children's), starting today.

Would you lose weight for Gold? In August 2013, Dubai offered its overweight residents a great incentive to drop kilos, one gram of gold for every kilogram lost. The 30 day weight loss plan was aimed at slimming down the local population, with obesity figures for that nation at 33%. The top three losers were also given a bonus of gold coins worth $5,400.

Chapter 2 – What is Lazy Loser?

I can't give Lazy Loser an official label or it will come off sounding like a diet, and then you will say, "Not another bloody diet book... that's all I need." Plus, I don't believe in diets so goodness knows I never would have created one. "Healthy-eating regime" doesn't take into account the love of my life - chocolate. Then there's "food plan", but that sounds like it involves a bit of work and organisation, and I'm too lazy for that.

What about "normal"? I think that best fits what I'm talking about. You could add many suffixes to it to make it more appealing: "Normal food", "normal eating", "normal chocolate binge", "normal drink or two", "normal life" — you get the idea. Actually, when you add "normal" to anything, it sounds easy and achievable. You think, *Ahhh yes, normal, I remember that — that was before Atkins, the soup diet, fasting, health shakes, detoxes, lycra leotards, and all the other hell I went through to drop a few kilos. Yes, I think I could handle normal.*

To me, when I add "normal" to "life", it doesn't mean boring or unimaginative. It suggests going through life without worrying about my health, weight, and food too much. Sure we're allowed to worry a bit about those things (I do), but what you eat and how much you exercise shouldn't be your biggest worry or the bane of your existence.

And don't get me started on the guilt. Why can't we just eat what we want and need, move enough to burn it off, and spend the rest of our time having fun? Surely that's not too much to ask for. OK, I can see the look on your face saying that's asking for the moon and stars — but really, it's not.

I'm often contacted by people asking me if they can join my Lazy Loser program. When I was living on the Sunshine Coast (now that I move around on tour, I run Lazy Loser online), I'd suggest a meet-up for a chat, usually at a coffee shop. Here's an example of what went down on the first Lazy Loser meeting (and no, I'm not just talking about the coffee and muffin, although that went down quite well too):

I'd ask questions along the lines of, "Why Lazy Loser?", "When and why did you start putting on weight?", "What have you done in the past to lose weight?" and so on. As you can imagine, the answers could be long, varied, and in some cases sad. I won't even attempt to recount them here, as that is a whole other book.

Then I ask four relevant questions that are the foundation of what Lazy Loser is about:

Question 1: *What is the number one thing you're doing in your life that is causing you to gain weight or not lose weight?*

Often, they'll start listing lots of reasons, so I try to get them to narrow it to one above all others.

Sitting can kill! A survey of 63,048 middle-aged Australian men who sat for more than four hours a day were significantly more likely to have a chronic disease like high blood pressure, heart disease, diabetes, or cancer. This was regardless of their body mass index (BMI), or how much they exercised when not sitting. Other studies show men who sit six hours a day are 20% more likely to die before men who sit for three hours a day. Women who sit for six hours a day are 40% more likely to die before their non-sitting counterparts.

I get many different answers to this: Drinking too much; having too many takeaway meals; over-snacking/grazing all day; going really well for a few days and then pigging out; and my favourite: Being a self-confessed chocoholic! The list goes on. Often, the main issues are general overeating, not being able to resist a certain food or drink, or laziness and inactivity. I prefer to get one definitive answer to this question, as it's a great base to kick off with. If I get lots of smaller answers or excuses or the big "I have no idea", it's harder, and I have to dig some more.

Lazy Loser Philosophy

If you're fat, that doesn't mean everything you're doing with your food intake or activity output is wrong or bad; about 70% of it is probably fine. However, more than likely, there are one or two weaknesses in your life that are causing you to put on weight or not lose it, and that is what you need to focus on. Why upend 70% of what you do and make unnecessary life changes when you can focus on one thing that is not quite right and change or adapt it? When you get a handle on that, maybe you can work on something else that has been an issue for you.

One of my favourite sayings is "Don't throw the baby out with the bath water", and that's the way I look at weight loss with Lazy Loser. Keep the baby (i.e. your healthy-food and good-exercise habits) and throw out the bath water (i.e. the small percentage of unhealthy things you're doing in your life).

Question 2: *Could you stop doing that thing or remove it from your life?*

This is when I get that cornered-rabbit look, with fear in their eyes.

"Don't panic," I say. "I'm not going to make you — I was just asking if you could."

Lazy Loser Philosophy

Why should you stop or remove anything you like to do (unless it's illegal, of course)? You probably could resist it for the short term — a week, or even a month. But boy, when you blow, you'll go back to that beloved habit and wallow in it like a pig in mud! And while you're depriving yourself of that love of your life, you'll obsess over it, crave it, dream of it, and even imagine your partner is a life-size version of it and try to gobble him or her up! All that torture only to go screaming back to your beloved food or drink and hide there for another month or longer, and the result? You get fatter.

Question 3: *What if I said you can have that yummy thing forever?*

Now the scared bunny has its ears pricked up.

Lazy Loser Philosophy

Wouldn't it be great if we could have the things we crave or obsess over the most in our lives? No, not Brad or Angelina (or both!) — we're talking food obsessions. So you don't have to give it up, and you know it's still there if needed. Think about it: Anything you love that becomes removed from your life, you miss. You don't think as much about things that are around you all the time, like partners, kids, or pets, but take those things away and you really notice that they are gone.

Question 4: *Would you be willing to make a deal with your yummy thing?*

The scared bunny gets that look of, "I'm listening..."

Lazy Loser Philosophy

A deal, a negotiation, a new strategy — isn't that what we do on a daily basis with ourselves, work, partners, family, kids and friends?

For example, you enjoy a couple of glasses of wine or beer after work. You can still have alcohol, but just one glass. Right away, you've cut your alcohol intake in half, which means half the calories and fat growth around your midsection. You love takeaway food

> **The hourglass figure is on its way out!** Only 8% of women have a true hourglass figure: Large bust, small waist, and curvy hips. In the 1950s, women's waists were smaller; on average, waists measured 70 cm (27.5 in.) and hips were a very curvy 99 cm (39 in.). The average woman's waist now measures 76 cm (32 in.), and we've shaved 7.5 cm of our hips down to 91.5 cm (36 in.). This is not a good thing, as it means we're changing from pears to apples — meaning women are carrying extra fat around their bellies.

and like to have it every weekend, you can keep the takeaway, but have it only once over the weekend, Saturday or Sunday — your choice — but not both days.

Then, the stunned bunny has the look of, "Hmmm, I smell a rat, what's the catch?" and replies with, "Wait a minute…I can't lose weight if I'm still drinking and eating rubbish, can I?"

I say, "You're gaining weight or not losing the weight you want, so surely halving the unhealthy food you're eating is going to have some impact on your weight, right?"

The scared, shocked, unsure, and slightly hopeful bunny then says, "OK, let's give this Lazy Loser thing a go."

That's it — really! This is what Lazy Loser is about.

It's not upending everything you've ever known and loved, not clearing out cupboards and fridges and throwing good food away. It's not going out and buying new shakes and bars and pre-packaged meals, or joining an expensive gym and then having to find the time to get there.

Lazy Loser looks at your normal life, puts it under a microscope, finds little things that don't need to be there, and shaves a few of them down to a normal size.

Lazy Loser Scales

Unless you've been residing on another planet until now, you should know that our weight is a product of the energy (food and drink) we put into ourselves against the energy output (all activity and exercise) we expend. This hasn't changed since Methuselah's day, and it's very unlikely it will change in our lifetime.

There is no magic bullet to weight loss. I wish there was and that it came coated in chocolate, but alas, there is not.

However, instead of bemoaning this fact, we should be happy – because it makes life uncomplicated. If we accept that it's as simple as "what goes in must come out in equal values", then we won't spend a lifetime and bucket of gold trying to chase theories from people telling us they've found that magic chocolate bullet.

I liken the energy-in, energy-out idea to old-fashioned weighted scales, with the plates on each end. One side holds all the food and drink we consume in a day, and the other side comprises the exercise and energy we expend in a day. If you're overweight, the food side is sitting on the counter and the energy side is swinging in the breeze.

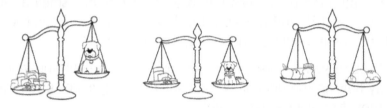

There is a very simple way to balance those scales: Take something from the food side, add something to the energy side, and keep this up over time until they are balanced. If you're happy with your weight, then your scales should be balanced forever, and you'll stay at the right weight for that length of time. Sure, the scales may tip a bit more to either side sometimes (e.g., when you have a big weekend, go on a holiday, or your mother cooks Christmas dinner), but those plates will balance again when you get back to your normal routine.

Lazy Loser is just that: A way to get the balance right. I gather my scales are balanced, as I haven't gone much over or under 65 kg in 17 years. That doesn't mean I am a health freak or eat like a bird — I got the balance right a long time ago, and now I know how to keep it there, by eating and moving (eat more = move more)!

Stop Getting Fatter

Balancing those scales is the most important thing you can do for your health. It means you'll stop putting on weight, and that is the very first point of Lazy Loser.

We don't wake up one day overweight or obese; we are getting fatter slowly. If you look back over the past 10 years and find you are 10 kg heavier, it means you have only put on one kilo a year.

One kilo in 365 days. That's one teaspoon of sugar a day, or one soft drink a week. Just think: If you eliminated those things 10 years ago, you wouldn't be overweight now. One less cup of tea or coffee a day (if you have sugar in it), one less drink a week ...

that sounds so easy that we could all do it and not even notice the difference.

Most people who start Lazy Loser are overweight, and are coming to me for help in losing weight. But I still maintain: Let's get the scales balanced first. Then when we're at the point where what we eat and how much energy we use is causing us to not gain weight, we can start adjusting the scales to tilt in the other direction. That, in turn, will result in weight loss.

If you're overweight and wanting to lose some kilos, the intake side of your scales needs to be higher in the air, with the energy-out side lower to the ground. If it stays that way for weeks or months, weight loss will happen — it has to. It means you're using more energy than you're eating. Eventually the scales will tip to balance, and then you're set for life. Keep the balance, and you'll stay in your healthy weight range.

"How long does it take to lose 10 kilos?"

This question, with some changes to the number of kilos, comes up at the end of the first Lazy Loser meeting and I have one answer. I stare the question asker down and say:

"It takes as long as it takes."

I never give timeframes or estimates of kilos you'll lose per week for the following reasons:

1. I'm too lazy to do the maths! I'm not prepared to count calories and then estimate how much exercise is needed to achieve a weekly weight loss. I prefer to start making changes to food and exercise patterns, monitoring those changes, and then making more alterations based on the results at the end of a week or month.

A study on the effects of sugar in rats found that rats fed a diet containing 25% sugar became anxious when the sugar was removed, displaying symptoms similar to people going through drug withdrawals, such as chattering teeth and the shakes.

2. You put on the weight — I didn't force feed you. So it's up to you to find out what made you fat, and how you can change that. I can help you work through it, but I'm not with you 24/7, so you need to tell me how much weight you want to lose and how you're going to do it.

3. We're all different. Our heights, weights, genders, lifestyles, and jobs all vary, and many of these things dictate how easy, hard, fast, or slow it is to drop weight.

Lazy Loser Rules

There aren't many, but Lazy Loser will not work without them;

Rule 1

Every day, you have to take something out of the left "energy-in/food and drink" side of your Lazy Loser scales and put something into the right "energy-out/exercise" side.

Examples:

• You normally have two poached eggs on two slices of buttered toast each morning. For Lazy Loser, you take out one slice of buttered toast (you won't even miss it) and add five extra minutes to your morning walk.

• You drink two stubbies of beer each evening after work. For Lazy Loser, you drop it back to one stubby, and decide to take the stairs at work instead of the elevator each day.

As you can see, Lazy Loser isn't asking for much — but both sides of your scales have to be tampered with, not just one. Adjusting both sides is a double whammy, and means you're eating less and doing more (so double the chance of losing weight).

Rule 2

When you take something out of the "energy-in/food and drink" side, you can't add anything new in.

For instance, in the examples above, you can't take out the piece of buttered toast and then think, *I might just stick a piece of bacon on the plate.* Or, when you cut back a stubby of beer at night, you can't say, "I'll have a can of Cola instead." This defeats the purpose of removing something.

Even if you think you could add a healthy food in, like an apple or something low in sugar like a Diet Cola, it's still a no-go. What is gone is gone, and not to be replaced. The only thing you can add to replace the food or drink you took out is water!

Lazy Bottom Line

• Lazy Loser is about finding the thing or things in your life that are causing you to put on or not lose weight, and changing or managing those things.

• Lazy Loser is not about cutting out the food or drink you love and crave — it's about making a deal with those things by having them around you, but not in the same quantities or as frequently.

• Lazy Loser is not about deprivation. As soon as you deprive yourself of anything you love — people, places, pets, and even food and drink — you want to be with them 10 times more, and they're all you can think about.

• Lazy Loser is like the old-fashioned weighted scales: Everything you eat and drink is on the left plate, and all your expended energy is on the right. If the left is on the ground, you're always going to be gaining weight. The objective is to balance the scales.

• Lazy Loser believes the first step is to stop putting on weight. When you have mastered that, make small changes to your diet and lifestyle to get on the road to losing weight.

• Monitoring energy-in and energy-out is the one and only way to manage weight. There are no magic solutions or food or pills to ever change this very basic formula. Accept it and start working on it.

• Once you determine the main factor causing you to gain weight or not lose it, deal with that thing only. If it's food or drink, halve the amount you normally have for a week, and see how that goes.

• Whenever you take something out of the left "energy-in/ food and drink" side of the scales, you can only add water to replace it — nothing else.

• You need to add something to your right "energy-out/ exercise" side of the scales every day. It doesn't have to be set exercise; just move more during the day. Five minutes more than usual is enough to start with.

• Visualise the scales, or even draw a picture of them. Draw one big picture of how they look at the moment, with all your daily food and drink on the left side and all your activity on the right. Then start crossing out or erasing on the left side and putting more on the right side, so you can see what is actually happening.

By 2025, 83 % of Australian men and 75 %of women 20 years and older will be obese or overweight based on current trends.

Chapter 3 – Fat Habits

Chapter 2 taught you the basics of how Lazy Loser works. Easy, isn't it? Figure out what you're doing wrong, change it, and you're on the road to weight loss and good health for life.

Yes, it would be great if it were that easy.

But (there is always one little but!) often the thing you need to change — whether it be a certain food or drink, a lack of activity, or a lifestyle issue — is one big bad habit that you need to break. This can be hard, but the good news is that they're all breakable.

I bet you've broken many habits during your lifetime. Think back over the years: There are probably many things that you did often and now don't do at all. Maybe you got tired of those things, found better things to do, or realised that those things were affecting your health and well-being — but you did change.

When I ask a Lazy Loser client about the one thing they're doing in their life that's causing them to gain weight or not lose it, I never hear an answer that isn't a habit.

Overeating, nibbling throughout the day, chocolate cravings, alcohol, binges, midnight munchies, sugary-drink obsessions, laziness: All habits and all can be broken.

There are two methods when it comes to breaking habits:

1. Cold turkey: Give it up altogether and then suffer, crave, and obsess over it every day for months.

2. Weaning: Slowly decrease the amount of, or the frequency you indulge in your habit.

I prefer the latter. I like to wean myself off my habit and find new options to take its place. Little changes are easier to handle; big changes are hard work.

Popular bad habits

Overeating at meal times

Habit: Somewhere along the path of life, you got used to large serving sizes. Often, we can blame our mothers for this, due to the way they insisted we eat every scrap on our plate, followed up with the mantra - "Think of the poor starving African kids" or the ultimate parental bribe - "If you don't eat it all you will go to bed without sweets".

When your stomach gets used to the idea of being full to the brim each time you eat, it grows, leaving more space to squish extra food in at your next meal. Overeaters have trained their tummies to store more each time. You're not overeating due to hunger and you're not naturally a big eater; you just got into the bad habit of loading too much food onto your plate, and then eating the lot.

Habit break: Start to decrease the amount of food you eat at mealtimes by dishing up what you would normally eat for one meal. Then divide everything (meat, vegetables, rice, pasta, etc.) into quarters and remove one quarter from the whole meal.

"What a waste," you say? Not really — move it onto someone else's plate, give it to the dog, or put it in the fridge for tomorrow's lunch.

In the United States, 90% of the money Americans spend on food is for the processed variety.

After you've finished your meal, monitor yourself to see if you feel hungry afterward. Chances are you'll feel as satisfied as you would have if you'd eaten that extra 25%. You don't have to dish the food up and then remove a quarter all the time — just until you get used to the idea of what your meal looks like at 75% size. After a while, you'll dish up the new, smaller amount automatically.

A similar method to reduce meal sizes is look at your normal-sized meal. How much of the plate does it cover? Is food hanging over the side, flush with the edge of the plate or top of the bowl?

If this is the case, take it back an inch (2.5 cm), so you see the edge of the plate or top of the bowl by that amount. This is a good visual tool when serving food.

If overeating at meals is your food habit:

• Never choose buffet meals or all-you-can-eat dinners.

• If someone else serves your meals, ask to dish your own food up (and explain why, so you don't offend your home chef).

• Never have second servings.

Snacking constantly between meals

Habit: This habit comes from having easy access to food. It often occurs with stay-at-home workers or parents, people who work in the food industry or are around food all the time. It can also be caused by not eating well and regularly at meal times. If you're putting something into your mouth within an hour of each meal, this is a bad habit, as it's not due to hunger.

Habit break: Remove yourself from the source or, if you can't do that, control your urges. Be pedantic about it — make sure you have a good, filling breakfast and set an alarm for yourself that goes off after two hours. Then you can have something to eat, but make it half a snack. This way you still get the snack that will feed your nibbling withdrawals, but you're taking something out of your left-hand intake scales. Remember: You're not hungry, so this snack is to make you feel better; a half snack will work just as well.

Set your snack alarm after each meal. If you're really struggling before your alarm goes off, distract yourself. Snacking often comes from boredom, so take a walk or perform another task at work instead of snacking.

If snacking or nibbling all day is your food habit:

• Don't buy snacks. If you have snacks in the house or at work, you'll crave and eat them.

• Change the type of snacks you eat. Make your snacks fresh fruit, so at least your snacking is healthy. If your usual snacks are high in sugar or salt this is a great way to break your cravings for those things as well.

• Halve the snack portions you'd usually eat.

• Don't miss out on meals; you'll snack all day if you miss breakfast.

Being addicted to high sugared food and drinks

Habit: Somewhere down the line, you got the taste for high-sugared foods, and now crave them constantly. The sugar habit is hard to break, because as we know, sugar is added to nearly everything we eat and drink. Don't stress about removing all sugar from your life, as it's not poisonous and won't kill you; however, too much will make you fat, and is not good for your health.

Habit break: Steering clear of processed foods, especially sweets, is the best way to break the habit. Even if you bake your own sweets or add sugar to your meals, that is still better and contains less sugar than processed foods. Don't drink your sugar — that's empty calories.

If you drink fizzy or sugary drinks daily, cut back to alternating days. Only drink water on the non-sugary-drink days. When you get used to the non-sugary-drink days (this could take a few weeks), cut your sugary-drink days to two per week. Finally, wean yourself to one day of sugary drinks, and you'll have broken your sugary-drink habit. Having a soft drink once a week as a treat is fine, so enjoy it.

Australia spends over $37 billion on fast food, making it the 11th biggest-spending fast-food nation in the world.

If sugar is your food habit:

• Cut your daily sugar intake in half: Halve sugary snacks or drinks, and use only half a teaspoon of sugar in tea and coffee instead of a full teaspoon.

• Steer clear of processed foods or, again, halve your intake of them.

• Swap your old snacks for fruit; fruit is still sweet and will give you the sugar hit, but cuts the cravings.

• Remove the sugar bowl from your house; you don't need it.

• Don't start the day with sugar, as you'll crave it all day. Ensure your breakfast has no added sugar.

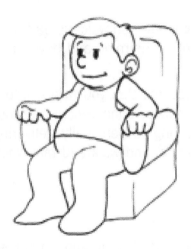

Being lazy

Habit: Believe or not, laziness is a habit. You're not born lazy; laziness is acquired. As a self-confessed lazy person, I see nothing wrong with being lazy. However, if you're overweight and sit in front of the TV for hours at a time, then laziness is your bad habit that needs changing. Watching TV is fine; it's the sitting while watching that's the problem.

Habit break: Don't give up your TV fix but, as with all Lazy Loser approaches, halve it. Pick the TV shows you must watch, and cut the ones that are not as important to you.

What do you do with your spare time? Move around! Turn the telly off an hour early, go to bed, and get up an hour earlier to exercise (there's nothing worth watching at 6 a.m.).

Can't give up your TV fix? Then give up the ads. Whenever a commercial comes on, leave the room. Walk up and down the stairs or grab your hand weights and do some resistance training.

Why not go out to the garage and bring in the old exercise equipment? An exercise bike and treadmill in front of the TV is perfectly fine: You're still watching, but moving at the same time. That is a win/win.

If laziness is your habit:

• Halve your laziness time. If you're sitting in front of the TV for four hours a night, do it for two hours; for the other two hours, move more.

• You don't have to exercise — just don't sit for long periods of time.

• Make a point of moving every hour of your waking day. In no time, getting up every hour and doing something will become a habit.

• If you're a lazy bones, go to bed earlier, so you wake up early and get going. You should feel fresher in the morning and have more energy.

• Think about each sitting activity you do. Can you turn it into a standing or walking activity? For instance, change some of your car sitting to walking; your office sitting to personally delivering messages inside or outside of the office; and walk and talk when you're on the phone.

Dieting habitually

Habit: Dieting is a very bad habit. Diets don't work, and when they end, you go back to your old ways: Eating a lot and getting fat. If you're one of those people who are always on a diet, you need to break that habit. It's bad for your health to change your eating and exercise patterns continually, and the highs and lows of this lifestyle can lead to self-loathing and unhappiness.

People with this habit often feel guilty when they're not on a diet; they need to convince themselves they are doing something to

Obese individuals sit 2.5 more hours a day than an individual of normal weight.

change their weight, and it becomes a vicious cycle. Nothing changes in their routine when the diet ends; it's an all-or-nothing approach.

Habit break: This one should be done cold turkey: Stop dieting! Tell yourself right now that you are never going on another diet. Habitual dieters need a new habit, as diets can be very addictive. You may hear or read of a new one and say, "Oh that sounds good, I'm going to try it out!" But first ask yourself, "Will I still be on this new diet in six months?" If the answer is no, then don't even go there. Eating packaged low-calorie meals, drinking diet shakes instead of eating, and leaving out important nutrients like carbs, protein, and fat are all signs of a diet program and it is never a solution to long term weight loss.

If you're a habitual dieter:

• Don't go on another diet.

• Look at what is making you put on weight: The answer is in your non-diet phase. Once you find that, start to change it.

• Steer clear of any diet or exercise routine that gives a timeframe (12-week challenge, six-week boot camp, four weeks to a bikini body, etc.). All of these things end — then what?

• If you can't break the diet habit, try designing your own diet (see Chapter 7: The Elephant in the Room).

• If you count calories, read labels, and weigh portions only when you're on a diet, then consider these things as diet habits and stop doing them; if you're doing something irregularly, it's not working for you.

Above are only some bad habits that can be broken, but there are plenty more. If your habit is not listed here, you may discover it later in this book, and find ways of adapting it or getting it out of your life for good.

The majority of a person's weight, obesity, and health woes are brought on by their lifestyles. If your bad habits have escalated to the point where they're affecting your ability to lose weight or be active, then that is a sign that you need to break them.

The best way to break a bad habit is to replace it with something else that is better for your health. Changing habits is easier, as the new thing is distracting and, after a while, becomes a new habit. This is when you'll forget why you were so hooked on your old habit.

However, try not to replace your old habit with a new food habit; just get rid of that eating habit. The best replacement is moving or exercising. This way, it's a double whammy: You're eating less and, with your new habit of moving more, stimulating more weight loss.

Old habit: Snacking at home.

New habit: Getting out of the house every hour (maybe gardening or go for a walk).

Old habit: Overeating at lunchtime.

New habit: Taking a smaller packed lunch to work and walking to the park to eat it.

Old habit: Drinking alcohol daily.

New habit: On your alcohol-free days, using the half hour or hour during which you'd normally drink to exercise.

Every time you think about the habit you're trying to break, get up and go for a 10-minute walk. By the time you're finished, the craving will be gone.

Lazy Bottom Line

- Understand that your weight gain or inability to lose weight is due to bad habits you've developed over time (from months to an entire lifetime).

- Habits are built into our systems and brains, but can be broken and changed.

- We often have several bad habits — work on changing one at a time; trying to change two at a time is too hard and likely to fail.

- Start with your worst bad habit. Begin chipping away at it little by little, day by day.

• Replace a bad habit with a good one: Swap sugary snacks with fresh fruit, halve your TV time with exercise time, etc.

• When you remove the bad habits, new habits will form. Make sure they're healthier than the habits you're getting rid of.

Physical inactivity is the fourth leading cause of death worldwide.

Chapter 4 – How Fat Are We?

How do we know when we're overweight or obese?

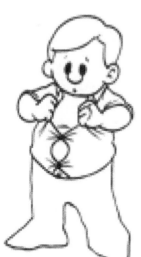

I would've thought bursting out of our clothes or going shopping and only just squeezing into XL or XXL sizes would be a tip off, but that's often not the case. Research shows most overweight or obese people underestimate their weight by 25%.

Believe it or not, being overweight or obese is not as obvious as you'd think — we need to be tested and told we are fat!

Every few months, articles in newspapers or on the internet tell us how fat we're getting as a nation. The results they quote are based on the body mass index (BMI) test. Scientists and doctors use BMI to classify our weight; however, I'm not happy with this classification.

BMI is calculated with the following equation:

BMI = (weight in kilos) / (height in metres X height in metres)

The BMI scale is as follows:

Underweight: Below 18.5

Normal: 18.5 to 24.9

Overweight: 25 to 29.9

Obese: 30 and higher

If you go by the BMI scale, half the professional rugby players are obese and the rest are overweight. Olympic weightlifters, boxers, basketball players, and many other top-level athletes have a BMI in the overweight or obese range.

BMI was introduced 200 years ago by a Belgian named Lambert Adolphe Jacques Quetelet. He produced the formula to give a quick and easy way to measure the general population's weight to assist the government in allocating resources.

However, when talking about BMI, there are some crucial points that should be noted:

Point 1: BMI is all about height.

BMI measures two factors: Height and weight. It doesn't take into account that humans are three dimensional, and that the third space is filled with a variety of things. BMI doesn't allow for body composition, body shape, or genetics. Muscle is a dense tissue; it weighs more than fat. Big, long, strong bones weigh more than short, weak bones. Even the size of a person's head can vary by kilos! All this means that a muscular, low-fat, strong-boned person will have a high BMI, and therefore be classified as overweight or obese.

Statistics tell us we're eating better and exercising more, but our national BMI growth says we're getting fatter. Are we just building muscle and strength, and therefore getting healthier in our heaviness?

A study of 17,000 people conducted in the U.S. found that those who sit for most of the day are 54% more likely to die of a heart attack.

We're growing up as well as out; our population is getting taller. When the BMI was invented 200 years ago, the average height of an Englishman was 170 cm (5'5"); an Englishwoman, 152 cm (5'). Australians' average height today is 176 cm (5'8") for males and 162 cm (5'3") for females.

On average, humans are growing taller and heavier. Between 1995 and 2012, the average height for men increased by 0.8 cm and for women by 0.4 cm, while the average weight for men increased by 3.9 kg and for women by 4.1 kg.

Our bones and the muscles attached to those bones are growing — which contributes to our higher BMIs.

Point 2: BMI does not differentiate between apples and pears.

The distribution of body weight, or more generally body shape, is a key predictor of health risk. It is now well established that individuals who deposit most of their body weight around their midsection (apple shape) are at much greater risk of disease and early mortality than people, who carry their weight more peripherally or below the hips (pear shape).

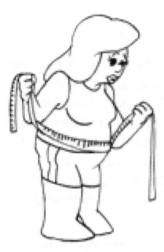

An easy way to check your risk is to measure your waist circumference. Current research suggests that a circumference of more than 94 cm in men and 80 cm in women shows an overweight level, while more than 102 cm in men and 88 cm in women denotes abdominal obesity.

A larger waist circumference can lead to a greater risk of diabetes, cardiovascular disease, mortality, and numerous other health problems. This suggests that waist circumference may be a more important measure of obesity and health risk than BMI.

Before you race away to get the tape measure, here are some guidelines:

• Measure directly against your skin.

• Breathe out normally.

• Make sure the tape is snug, without compressing the skin.

• The correct place to measure your waist is horizontally halfway between your lowest rib and the top of your hipbone. This is roughly in line with your belly button.

In Australia in 2012, 60.3% of men and 66.6% of women 18 years and older had a waist circumference that put them at an increased risk of developing chronic disease.

Point 3: What about fat?

We usually know when we've put on a few kilos: We can see it, feel it, and pinch it; our clothes are tighter, and we don't feel as fit or energetic. In case you didn't know: Those wobbly bits are fat!

But fat isn't just on the outside — visceral fat lines our organs and blocks our blood vessels. This is the dangerous fat! If your body fat is too high, you put yourself at risk of getting some of the common health problems we face today. High blood pressure and cholesterol, diabetes, obesity, and some cancers can be due to high levels of body fat.

A certain amount of fat is essential to bodily functions. It regulates your body temperature, protects and insulates organs and other tissues, and is the main form of the body's energy storage. However, the essential fat range for women is around 10 to 12%, and for men only 2 to 4%.

Body-fat readings are very important in knowing your true health, inside and out. Not all overweight people have a high percentage of body fat, and not all skinny people have a low one. Active people who are constantly moving or regularly exercising burn more fat, so even though they may weigh more, their body-fat readings could be in the recommended range. Similarly, thin people who don't exercise and eat a high-fat, high-sugar diet may be sitting on the very high side and not even be aware. People of the same height and weight can have largely varying body compositions.

People who sat more than 11 hours a day have a 40 % higher risk of dying within three years.

The human body is made up of many different tissues; mostly water, bone, lean tissue, and adipose tissue (fat). When we talk about body-fat percentage it is just that: The amount of fat in our bodies. However, it is not just the chubby skin fat we can pinch — it is also made up of visceral fat.

The way I measure the body fat of my clients is with the bioelectrical impedance analysis (BIA) scales. I use this method because it's easy, less invasive, and cheaper than other methods. When done regularly it can give you an idea of how your body-fat levels are going.

In general terms, BIA is a small electric current that is sent through the body (in the scales' case, through the feet). The resistance to the electrical stimulus is different when it encounters fat, lean muscle, and skeletal tissue.

Muscles are a good electrical conductor, as they have a high percentage of water; however, fat is a poor conductor. Some inaccuracies with the BIA are due to the amount of water you've consumed prior to weighing or your general hydration levels. As electrical currents travel better through water, more fluid may give you a lower body-fat reading.

Readings can also be affected by alcohol, caffeine, eating or exercising prior to testing, and, for women, the time of the month. The best time to do the BIA is in the morning before eating, drinking, or exercising.

You will notice in the charts below that men are required to (and often do) have a lower body fat percentage than women. This is because women carry more adipose tissue in the body. Women's breasts are all adipose tissue, and they carry more fat around their hips as well. Men have bigger muscles, and therefore the percentage of muscle mass should be more than fat.

You'll also notice in the charts that the older we get, the more body fat we're allowed to have and still remain in the healthy range. Visceral (internal) fat increases, and our muscle mass decreases with age.

My goal in life is to always be in the recommended range, and at 50, I still am. I'm aiming to keep it there for 50 more years!

You should know your body fat levels. Basic scales can give you a reading, and although it will be a general reading, it will still give you an idea of where you are on the body-fat scale. True readings of body-fat levels are done by being weighed underwater (or an embarrassing skin-fold test can be accurate as well).

The charts below display body-fat ranges by gender and age:

FEMALE

Age	20-29	30-39	40-49	50-59	60+
Very High	>39	>40	>41	>42	>43
High	33-39	34-40	35-41	36-42	37-43
Recommended	17-33	18-34	20-35	22-36	24-37
Below Av.	12-17	13-18	14-20	15-22	16-24
Low	<12	<13	<14	<15	<16

MALE

Age	20-29	30-39	40-49	50-59	60+
Very High	>25	>28	>30	>32	>35
High	20-25	22-28	25-30	27-32	30-35
Recommended	15-20	17-22	18-25	20-27	22-30
Below Av.	8-15	10-17	11-18	12-20	15-22
Low	5-8	6-10	7-11	8-12	9-15

Point 4: Consider all the other stuff we can't see.

Cholesterol is a fatty substance in our blood that can line and block the arteries, but we can't see or feel it from out here! Our blood could be struggling to get through or circulate to all areas of our body. Often we don't even know, and BMI is not going to tell us that.

Smell the roses! Researchers at Harvard conducted a behavioural survey; the results showed that if people saw fresh flowers in the morning, they had more energy during the day!

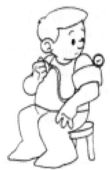

We can't see or often feel our blood pressure, but high blood pressure is an important risk factor for heart disease, stroke, and other cardiovascular diseases. According to WHO (World Health Organisation) guidelines, a person is defined as having high blood pressure if his or her systolic or diastolic pressure is greater than or equal to 140/90 mmHg.

In 2012, just over 3.1 million Australian people 18 years and older (21.5%) had measured high blood pressure. Overall, men were more likely to have higher blood pressure readings than women (23.6% and 19.5%, respectively), while the proportion of Australians with high blood pressure increased with age.

Blood-pressure charts

There are two figures on the blood-pressure score:

1. The systolic number (top-line) is the reading when the heart contracts and pushes the blood through the arteries.

2. The Diastolic number (bottom-line) is the reading when the heart is resting between beats.

Hypertension is the name given to high-blood-pressure.

	Systolic	Over	Diastolic
Normal	120	/	<80
Pre-hypertension	120-139	/	80-89
High blood pressure (hypertension stage 1)	140-159	/	90-99
High blood pressure (hypertension stage 2)	>160	/	>100
Emergency hypertension	>180	/	>110

So how fat are we?

When it comes to health and testing, there's a process you need to go through to make sure you're fit, healthy and disease-free:

1. Be aware of your BMI.

2. Know what your body-fat reading is, and check to see what range you're in. If it's high, work on getting it into the recommended range by following Lazy Loser.

3. Find out if your waist circumference is within a healthy range.

4. Know your body shape. More than likely, it's similar to one of your parents' and cannot be changed; but remember, obesity is not a body shape.

5. Get a blood-pressure reading and find out if you have a family history of high blood pressure, stroke, and/or heart disease.

6. Have your doctor order a blood test for your cholesterol levels, and find out if you have a family history of high cholesterol.

7. If you are overweight, obese, or have a family history of diabetes, get your blood-sugar levels tested. Your doctor or pharmacist can do this simple test.

8. Speak to a doctor, nurse, or pharmacist to find out any other information that may be able to help you on your health journey.

New Yorkers live an average of nine months longer than other U.S. citizens. Since 1980, Big Apple residents have increased their lifespans by 6.2 years compared to the 2.5 years of the rest of the nation. The rates of heart disease and cancers are dropping more in New York than any other city. Why? They walk. New Yorkers walk more than the average American, and they walk faster; studies show that they are the fastest walkers in the country. Other studies show that people who live in urban centres weigh an average of 5 kg less than their suburban or country counterparts. This is known as the urban health advantage.

But wait — there's more.

What about our fat perception?

Okay, now you know all the facts about fat, size, and health inside and out. But often that means nothing if we just feel fat or can't zip up our favourite jeans.

Bottom line: Looking good and fitting into a certain size is what most people want from losing weight. Forget the health and fitness — you just want to squeeze into those skinny jeans!

We want to look like the people we see in magazines, on TV, and in movies. We would like their bums, boobs, noses, and hair (and their pay cheques would be okay as well).

What about reality? It's the thing society is losing touch with, and it's often a bigger problem than our chubby thighs.

I have met women in their thirties with a few kids in tow who tell me they want to fit into a size 6 or 8. I ask them if they've ever worn those mini sizes and they say no, but that it is their dream. I often think, Dream on.

Is it realistic to be a size and shape you've never been, or furthermore, a size and shape none of your family or ancestors have ever been?

I do many health-and-fitness assessments, and am often shocked by the answers I get when I ask the people standing in front of me what they want to get out of the fitness program they're signing up for.

I've had women prefer to show me how they want to look — not with their own wedding or pre-children photos, but with glossy magazine cut-outs of stick-thin catwalk models. I usually say, "So, you want to grow three feet taller, be pre-pubescent (as this girl is about 13), and have a touch-up artist with you at all times?"

My sarcasm doesn't go down very well, but I have to be honest. The likelihood of any of us looking like a catwalk model is very, very slim (pardon the pun). But more importantly, why would you want to? Is being stick thin going to make your life better, happier, or more fun?

Don't answer that, I will: No, it won't!

Being a weight you can live with and wearing sizes and clothes you've worn before that felt comfortable and you've looked good in are the best goals to have. Why? Because they're achievable — as you've been there and done that, you can get back there again.

Trying to look like someone else or be a weight or size you've never been is either not possible for you or too hard to achieve — meaning you'll fail, and most likely always be fat.

To be successful at losing weight, you have to change those unrealistic goals and images you have in your head. Set your own goals for a weight that is right for you.

Here are my suggestions to get you started:

1. Start by managing the weight you're at now. Look back and think about when you started to put on weight, how much you've gained, and why you gained it. Was it after you had a baby; when you changed jobs; did you have an injury or illness that meant you couldn't exercise? If you think hard, you'll find the answer. Knowing what caused it is a good thing, because then you can figure out how to change it. And while you can't change the reason, you can stop blaming it, adjust, and move on.

2. Make your first goal to stop putting on weight.

3. Set up a Lazy Loser program for yourself: Take something out of the left side of your scales (energy-in/food and drink) and add something to the right side (energy-out/exercise).

4. Follow Step 3 for a few weeks and see what happens.

5. Adjust the scales again: Remove some more unhealthy food-and-drink habits from the left side and add a few extra energy minutes into the right.

6. Repeat Step 5 until you lose 5 kg (no timeframe — just keep at it).

7. Want to lose more than 5 kg? Repeat steps 3 to5.

I know, I can hear you: "That will take forever!"

Well great, because you have forever — and that is a good thing to have on your side. If it takes a lifetime, it means you have done the right thing and are improving your health for life.

(P.S. It won't take forever.)

Lazy Tale

I was a fat child and teenager.

How fat? I don't know. Ask my brothers: They used to call me "Fatty Boombah", and constantly ask, "When is your baby due?" My mum used to counteract their taunts with, "Leave her alone; it's only puppy fat," to which they would reply, "Oh great, she must be due to have a Labrador any day now."

Ha ha. Don't you just love brothers?

When you read "Chapter 6: The Skinny Sister-in-Law", you may relate. I do, as I was living in a house full of skinnies: Three were tall, beanpole boys and one was a tall, thin girl. I don't know how fat I was, but in that house I was enormous, and felt like the fattest person who ever lived.

When I went to secondary school, I met a new friend, and we became inseparable for six years. She was a little chubby, but not as fat as me (remember: I was the fattest person in the world). She was very confident about her weight, and never gave the impression that she was ever worried about it.

During our years of friendship, I spent my time trying to cover every spare inch of flesh with the biggest, baggiest clothing I could find — if only I realised that the tents I was wearing made me look larger than I really was. But my best buddy had no problems showing off as much flesh as she could — her school skirts were shorter than school rules allowed; she exposed her midriff on every possible occasion; and while she wore teeny tiny bikinis on the beach, I had a huge T-shirt on to hide my ugly one-piece.

My friend had four siblings as well, but they were different from my family. Two of her sisters and one brother were overweight, and her mum was obese. In her family, she was told how thin and pretty she was, and often encouraged to eat another slice of pie, as she was getting too thin!

The year of our debutante ball, we tried out a new "Bikini-Body Diet" that was highlighted in a teen magazine so as to look our absolute best on the big night. She came over to my place to have an official weigh in. She stepped on the scales first: 62 kg popped up. Then it was my turn. I stepped on gingerly (didn't want to break the scales), and then my reading came up: 62 kg.

I was gobsmacked. How could my confident, bikini-wearing friend weigh the same as me? I could tell she was just as shocked; how could she be as heavy as her fat friend? We put it down to my scales being dodgy and never mentioned our weights again!

I now realise that fat is different in everyone's eyes. How we feel about our bodies; compared to what we see in the mirror; the way others view us; the attitudes of the people we live with; and the comments people make, tell us more about how fat we are or feel than the numbers on those horrid bathroom scales.

Lazy Bottom Line

• Don't get caught up in the media hype about obesity as ranked by BMI. You are an individual, and need to know a lot more about your own weight before you classify yourself as overweight or obese from your BMI.

• Find out what your body-fat reading is; it's a good indicator of overall health.

• If you're overweight and unfit, go to the doctor for a check-up. Get your blood-pressure, cholesterol, and blood-sugar levels checked. Tell your doctor you want to lose weight; he or she will help and support you.

• Be realistic. Aim to lose weight to get back to a size you've been as an adult. Find a favourite piece of clothing you once wore that no longer fits, and make your first goal to get back into it. You were there once, so you can get back there again.

• Don't set timeframes or weekly weight-loss goals. Not putting on weight is a great start, and losing a little is fantastic. Every week is different, and often our lifestyles and moods go up and down, as does our weight.

• Try not to focus as much on the kilos you lose, and instead gauge your success on the way you feel. Do you feel fitter, stronger, healthier, and happier? I'd rather lose a gram and feel fitter and happier than lose two kilos and feel hungry and flat!

• Take your time – Lazy Loser is a project for you to live a long healthy life and hopefully that is a long, long time.

In 1949, the average consumption of butter in Australia was 11 kg per person; 50 years later, it's 4.1 kg. In 1949, we ate only half a kilo of margarine yearly; now we consume an average of 4 kg.

Chapter 5 – Big Fat Excuses

These are the excuses I hear, and the responses below are the thoughts I have when I hear them:

I have the fat gene.

Yeah, your parents are fat...so?

My metabolism is slow.

It's slow because you're too lazy to move more.

I've tried everything and nothing works — I just put on weight!

Just a thought: have you tried eating less and moving more?

It's my hormones.

Maybe, but are you medically qualified to make that diagnosis?

I'm big boned.

It's the padding around those bones that's the problem.

I eat like a bird and still can't lose weight.

Maybe Big Bird from "Sesame Street".

I'm not in the right frame of mind at the moment to lose weight.

Oh, is Right Frame of Mind on a holiday? When do you expect him back?

I know it sounds harsh; being overweight is a sensitive issue, which is why my responses are in my head. I try and soften the blow when I address each statement, but basically they're all excuses when it comes to losing weight.

First things first

Losing weight doesn't come easily to most people. I agree with that, and am sympathetic. When clients come to me asking for my help in losing weight, I'm their best buddy. I think it's fantastic they are realising that their weight and current lifestyle are issues, and are attempting to change that and get healthy.

However, when I sit down and talk to people who are interested in becoming Lazy Losers, I invariably hear the above excuses. I let them know from the get-go that if they really believe those things, they shouldn't bother starting a new eating or fitness program.

I tell them they will fail, because they've already written their excuse. If it fails on week one, they can say, "See, I told you — I've tried everything, and it always fails." (For the record, one week doesn't qualify as trying.) If it fails on week four, they can say, "My pesky fat gene won't let me lose weight."

If you have your excuse script ready, then failure is guaranteed.

To succeed, you need to clear the excuses from your mind and start with a fresh slate. The best thing to write on that slate is:

I am overweight, and I need to lose weight to make me healthier and happier.

That's it — no "but"s, no post-mortems, and no past excuses.

The fat gene

"I know what my problem is: My obesity is genetic. Mum's obese and riddled with arthritis. Dad was fat until he had a heart attack and lost 50 kilos; now he's a fitness fanatic and it drives Mum mad. Auntie Jean is enormous. My grandparents were really skinny, but that's just because they grew up in the depression and times were tough. My youngest is chubby, so I think he's going to take after me."

This is a real statement from a Lazy Loser, and while I was listening, I was thinking, "Wow. Not only have you written your own excuses, but you've got plenty to go around the family as well."

Is there a fat gene?

I'm not going to say there isn't, as I don't know, but the jury is out among the people who should know (researchers, scientists, and academics). And if the jury is out, then we officially have to stop using the fat-gene excuse until the evidence in irrefutable.

There is no height gene that makes us tall, so there's not likely to be a fat gene that makes us obese. However, there may be a series of genetic links that could, when they contain a fat style of gene, affect the way people store and use the energy they consume. However, even if there is, it would affect less than 2% of the people who are obese. So what excuses are the other 98% going to use now?

Scientists say when they can accurately pin down that pesky gene, they'll work on finding a drug to help counter the effects of it — but the drug is a good 10 years off. Well, looks like we'll just have to kick back, eat and drink, and wait. And if we haven't dropped dead by then from diabetes or heart disease, let's take that fat antidote and get on with living our healthy, wonderful lives!

Most scientists also ask that even if fat genes are running around inside us or there's one big fat gene directing all our eating, is it worth testing for? Diet and exercise are relevant regardless of what they discover, so lifestyle changes will still be the main area to re-evaluate.

Genes can be hit and miss and some of us are not doled out the best lot, but we all make do with what we have. We get on in the world, study, work, fall in love, reproduce, and have fun despite

The U.S. has the highest daily consumption of calories in the world per person — they average 3,770 calories a day — yet only 6.9 % of their annual income is spent on food. The lowest consumption of calories is in the Democratic Republic of the Congo, with an average of 1,500 calories — and they have to spend 50 % of their income on food.

our differing genetic makeups. People who are unlucky enough to be slapped with a disease gene from birth tend to be real fighters; they know what they're up against and try to lead the best lives they can, all while coping and dealing with their flawed genetic imprints.

So if you were one of a rare few who did get slapped with the fat gene, you too would not just lie down and let it be — you'd get up and fight on.

Regardless of the breakthrough technologies in finding fat genes, researchers still lay the blame for the obesity epidemic on lifestyle. We eat too much and move too little. We sit for longer amounts of time and eat more than we ever have in history.

Feel like blaming it on Mum and Dad? Go for it. If your mum and dad were fatties, they didn't get that way by eating fruits and vegetables and running marathons; they got that way by eating unhealthily and not exercising enough. You lived with them, they brought the food they ate into the house, and you had to eat it; you had no choice. They wouldn't take you out bike riding or walking and you couldn't go by yourself, so you grew up fat and lazy with no idea of how to change the cycle. Blame them now; in fact, take 10 minutes to blame them in your head.

Now STOP. Move forward. You are an adult now, and the best thing about being a grownup is not having to do what your parents tell you to do, ever again. You are in charge, and if you go through the rest of your life as fat as your parents and die young because of it, they are not to blame — you are. The buck stops with you now. The weight you carried around as a child or teenager can be removed; it doesn't have to stay there forever.

While we are on the topic of the Blame Game, there are a few other things we can sling mud at:

• The huge multinational companies that keep producing fatty, tasty, unhealthy food and shoving it in our faces at every turn through crafty marketing and advertising.

• The diet companies that suck you in and make promises. You believed them, threw money at them, followed their programs to the letter, lost the weight, and then stacked it back on again.

• The school tuck shop or university cafeteria that served up unhealthy crap day after day. You enjoyed every morsel, but now you're fat because of it.

These are all worthy nominees to lay blame on. But that's in the past. If you fall into their traps now, then you are to blame, as you know the rules and how to break them. Every skerrick that goes in your mouth now is your call; every bit of movement you do to burn it off is in your control.

Metabolism

Metabolism describes the chemical processes occurring within a living cell or organism that are necessary for the maintenance of life. The term is commonly used to refer specifically to the breakdown of food and its transformation into energy.

That is a very simplistic definition of a quite complicated process, but the word, like many health buzz words, often gets bandied about with a negative connotation about poor diet and exercise: "I have a very slow metabolism, so losing weight is a lot harder for me." In a way that person is right — if he or she is carrying lots of fat and less muscle, then yes, the metabolism is slower. But that's not the metabolism's fault — it's the person's fault for eating too much and exercising too little.

Everyone has a different metabolism, just as everyone's resting metabolic rate is different. Resting Metabolic Rate (RMR) is the rate in which you burn calories when doing absolutely nothing (even when you're chilling out on the couch, you're burning calories). Simply being alive — breathing, growing, hormone production,

Coca-Cola reports average per-capita consumption by country of the company's drinks, including their bottled waters, sports drinks, and various sodas. The figures are based on a serving size of 8 oz (240 ml). Number of servings per year: India: 12, China: 38, Kenya: 40, Russia: 73, South Korea: 84, France: 149, Japan: 179, Germany: 190, Great Britain: 210, Brazil: 230, South Africa: 247, Canada: 259, United States: 403, Mexico: 728.

inner temperature regulation, thinking (yes, using your brain!) — burns calories. However, since everyone's RMR is different, they burn calories at different rates.

One way to lower your RMR (meaning make it slower and unable to burn calories as effectively) is — surprise — to diet. The more you deprive yourself of food, the more your body panics; it thinks starvation is coming and that it's time to protect your fat reserves. The way your body does this is by slowing your metabolism to store the calories you consume. Yo-yo dieting, which is common among dieters, gets your body to a point where it thinks, I'm saving some of the fat, as you never know when this crazy person is going to starve me again!

Here's a breakdown of how we burn calories:

RMR burns a whopping 60-70% of all the calories you eat, so just doing nothing still means the inner workings of the body are hard at it — breathing, heartbeat, growing, temperature regulation, and thinking burns most of our daily calories.

Eating burns another 10%; just chewing, munching, crunching, and digesting burns 10% of your daily calories.

The other 30% comes from exercise, an active lifestyle, and incidental activity; this is the area we can have some control over to change the way our metabolism works.

As you can see, most of your calories are burned from doing nothing — or should I say living!

Unfortunately, fad diets and supplement companies solely blame slow metabolism for weight gain. Overweight people have quickly picked up on this, and use the slow-metabolism card as just another excuse to explain their weight. Many people blame a slow metabolism on low thyroid function, age, and hormones, when really these things have very little impact on it. The major impact is muscle, and the amount of muscle you have often dictates a slow or fast metabolism.

Certain parts of your body burn more calories than others, and muscles burn a lot more calories than fat. In fact, a kilo of muscle burns between 120 and 150 calories per hour, whereas a kilo of fat burns fewer than 10 calories per hour; that's a big difference.

This is one of the reasons men are allowed more daily calorie allowances than women — they have more muscle.

Another misconception about muscle and fat is that people think they're connected, as if muscle turns into fat when not used and fat can be converted to muscle. Wrong again; they're two very different types of tissue, and do not morph into each other. Fat people do have muscles; maybe they're not as big or as toned, but they're there. They're just lying under the fat, and therefore not seen or even felt when flexed. Reducing the fat layer and increasing the muscle mass by exercise or resistance training is the way we eventually see and feel the muscle.

Weight loss is great if that's your goal and changing what you eat or not overeating is the best. But don't discount the importance of exercising to work on increasing your muscle mass, which stimulates metabolism.

There are other factors that dictate a slow or fast metabolism:

• **Muscle mass.** As I said above, this is the major factor that sets your metabolic rate.

• **Eating frequency.** Eating smaller meals regularly helps speed up metabolism. As discussed above, going a long time between eating suggests to your body there is a famine coming, and it goes into a slight shutdown. This is one of the reasons breakfast is very important in speeding up metabolism — it breaks the night-time fast, and gets your metabolism kick-started first thing in the morning.

• **Activity level.** This refers not just to exercise, but to your job's activity level and all your incidental exercise.

• **Food choices.** Low-fat or low-carb diets that make you feel weak or hungry between meals don't boost your energy levels, and therefore do nothing for metabolism growth.

• **Diet and exercise fads.** Your body takes a while to adapt to new things, and once it has, it starts to gain benefits and health can be improved. But continually starting diet and exercise fads and then going off them for weeks or months confuses all your systems. Consistency with diet and exercise will gradually give you the correct metabolism for life. The ultimate goal to a healthy life is to be within the correct height/weight/body fat range and stay there — forever. Sure it may fluctuate on occasion (like holidays or special celebrations), that's fine as long as you know it only takes a bit of extra exercise and cutting back on some foods to get on track.

Another misconception with metabolism is that metabolism slows down with age. Once again, we're blaming something that only changes when other factors come into play. Instead of blaming your slow metabolism when you're older, consider that maybe you're overeating or eating too much of the wrong foods and moving less than you used to.

Older people are less likely to be still part of high energy team sports, like football, netball, or tennis. Although they may still exercise, it's not at the same intensity as it was when they were younger. Family life changes when we get older; parents chase after toddlers and school children for years and do more household chores, they cut back on those activities when the kids grow up. Therefore, it still comes back to lifestyle. You've cut back on certain activities over time, but you still eat the same, that is the cause of your middle age spread, not metabolism. This is an important time of your life to have a good hard look at your Lazy Loser scales and tweak them.

I've tried everything, and nothing works!

This is a tough one, as I'm sure most people who struggle with their weight have had a go at fads, crazes, and even healthy-eating regimes and found it very frustrating to see that it worked for only a short time until the weight crept back on.

However, the weight only crept back on after you'd finished the new diet or eating or exercise program — not while you were on it.

Close to 220,000 Americans have weight-loss-surgery operations annually —a sevenfold leap in a decade, according to industry figures — costing more than $6 billion a year.

This shows the obvious: When you go back to your old ways, you get fat again. It's your old ways that are making you fat, not the new ways.

Change your old ways. But keep in mind that anything requiring a total overhaul of what you're doing now is destined to fail for two reasons:

1. It's not natural to you.

2. You don't like it that much.

You won't do anything that you don't like for very long; this is true for most things in life. Effort takes commitment; have you got what it takes? Overhauling everything you eat and drink is challenging. And if you're lazy like me, you may not be up to such a big challenge.

Believe it or not, your old ways are probably not so bad — it's true! Sure, there are some things in there that are out of whack and not working for you, but I bet 70% of what you're doing is okay.

Therefore, instead of the overhaul, just work on the 30% that isn't working for you. The 30% could be your food choices, lack of activity, or both, so change that. Alter some of your food habits and add 30% more activity to your life (even if you do minimal activity now, 30% is still more than that). That's a 60% turnaround, so it has to work.

Some weeks you may fall off the wagon and only change 10% of your energy-in, energy-out formula. That's still a change, and it all adds up. No, not as fast as the celery and water diet, but it's far healthier and easier to live with.

So when you say you've tried everything, have you tried my normal method? If it's the one last thing you try, please have a go.

Hormones

Research does show that hormone levels vary over our lives and can get out of whack and affect the way we crave, process, and burn foods. However, before you yell, "I told you my hormones are the cause of my big bum!" realise that no they're not — you are still the cause of your large posterior.

Diets, especially crash diets that deprive the body and brain of the levels of nutrients and energy they need, cause our hormones to panic and start to react. Fatigue and lethargy sets in. Any exercise we do doesn't burn the calories, as the body is hanging on to them for dear life. It works the same if you've been eating a high-sugar and high-processed-food diet for many years: Your body sets the hormone insulin on a sweet rollercoaster ride with lots of highs and lows, but not much weight loss.

So yes, hormones play a part. They're the body's inbuilt regulators, but are they making you fat? NO. The ridiculous diets and eating regimes you've done in the past, the fits and spasms you have at exercising, and the levels of sugar you put into your mouth are the cause, which still makes your lifestyle the culprit.

Does this mean you can't change your hormones? NO again. You trained your hormones to be erratic; you can train them to change back to normal.

The bottom line on hormones is: Are they really out of whack?

When a Lazy Loser client gives me the hormone excuse, the first thing I say is:

"Did your doctor diagnose that your hormones are causing your weight gain?"

"Oh no," they reply. "I just know they are."

"How do you know?" I ask. I get a range of answers about how they feel fatigued or flat. Women tell me they have had erratic or irregular periods, are going through the change, have had trouble with losing weight in the past, or have read a book titled something like "The Killer Hormones". Many hormone problems are self-diagnosed.

If you think you have an issue with your hormones, go to a doctor, who will order some tests and tell you once and for all if that's your real problem. The good thing is that if the tests show hormone inconsistences, then you're on the right path and they can be treated. And believe it or not, often a healthy diet-and-exercise program is the first thing prescribed.

Big bones

This is a funny one, because how can we ever know whether we have large bones? Doctors can't exactly strip off your skin, weigh and measure your skeleton, and give you a big-bone diagnosis. Besides, it's not the bones that are the worry — it's what those bones are padded with, which is more than likely a lot of fat.

I know I'm being blasé about the big bones, but this excuse is more related to overall size and shape. And you'd likely be right if you told me you have a solid or heavy build. We see all the wonderful body shapes and sizes everywhere.

We know some people are petite, small-framed, and tiny; this applies to both sexes. And then we have tall, solid (not fat), statuesque builds in both males and females.

However, the petites are not always skinny or underweight and the statuesque are not always fat or overweight, even though their weights may vary dramatically. It's true that the taller you are and the more muscle tissue you have, the heavier you are. And yes, your bones may be bigger and longer (and as a result, heavier as well), and that is not fat or unhealthy.

Fat is the rolls and folds you feel and see. And while altering your unhealthy food choices won't make you lose weight off your big bones, it will take off some of the pressuring fat that is padding and stopping them from moving as effectively. The greatest thing about exercise is that it strengthens your bones, so you'll have big strong ones — the best kind to have!

I eat like a bird!

I'm not sure what amount birds eat, but by the size of most of them, I'm guessing not much. This statement often refers to eating small amounts but staying fat or not being able to lose weight.

Who jumps on the scales the most? The French weigh themselves the most (every day). Singaporeans weigh themselves the least.

In essence, this can be true as well. You may eat small servings and not as much as other people you know who are thinner than you. However, if those small meals are laden with sugar and fat or washed down with litres of high-calorie drinks, then the bird will turn into a big one.

Instead of focusing on the amount you eat, pay attention to what you eat. With weight loss, you have to account for everything that goes into your mouth — not just what's on your plate at meal times. It's the type of milk that's in your three lattes a day, the non-water drinks you consume, the mints on your desk that you eat mindlessly, the complimentary nuts you had at the bar with your beer, the leftovers you're clearing up after dinner, and so on. Many people who say they don't eat much have blinders on to all the food and drink that is consumed outside of mealtimes. It's more than likely these foods that are making you fat.

Right frame of mind

This statement really gets my goat! Let me offer you some similar statements people have tried using on me about their health and fitness over the years:

"I'd like to get fitter but I'm just not in the right headspace at the moment."

Translation: I don't want to get fitter.

"I'm really overweight and I'm going to go on a diet when I'm in the right frame of mind."

Translation: I'm fat and lazy, and I just can't be bothered trying to lose weight.

"I'd like learn how to run, but I have to get my head around it first."

Translation: I don't want to be a runner.

I know many psychologists will be hunting me down, saying that being in the right frame of mind is important before you take on anything major in your life. However, I don't buy it!

My very simple philosophy is: If you want to do something, **you will**, and if you don't, **you won't**.

People refer to "Right Frame of Mind" as though it's another entity they have no control over. But it's your frame of mind and you own it. You're just giving yourself another excuse to not do what you've been putting off.

I've also noticed the "Right Frame of Mind" statement only applies to things you're not keen to do, or something that puts you out of your comfort zone. For example, I don't often hear, "I can't face that last slice of pizza because I'm not in the right headspace" or "I can't look at that box of chocolates at the moment; my frame of mind isn't right."

Stop blaming your head for not making changes to your life or creating some great challenges for yourself.

You want to lose weight? Make the changes now. You can start your Lazy Loser regime right away, and if your head is saying I can't get around this, tell it to get on board or it will get left behind!

Lazy Bottom Line

• If you think you have sure-fire reasons why you're overweight, they may be true, but are all ultimately excuses?

• Putting on weight is extremely easy, and losing it is very hard. That is a fact, and you can use that. But don't turn it into something that says it's not possible or hopeless; it can be done.

• If you think there's something biological stopping you from losing weight, visit the doctor and get a diagnosis, find the cure, and work toward it. Half the battle is knowing what the problem is — then you can work on fixing it.

• Be honest with yourself; it's no good lying to or cheating the most important person in your life. Take a good hard look at what you eat and how you burn off your food. If you're overweight, the solution will be in that equation; like all mathematical problems, there's a correct answer. But you won't find the answer if you're fudging the figures.

• We all come in differently shaped packages; even babies are born small and petite or big and roly-poly. Be proud of your build and natural shape. However, realise it's not the shape and structure of your body that is the problem if you're overweight — it's the fat that is padding out that shape and structure. That fat is one thing you can change and remodel.

Chapter 6 – The Skinny Sister-in-Law

We all have one (or a relative or friend) — and if you can't find one in your circle, maybe you're it!

The reason I say "skinny sister-in-law" is because of a story one of my Lazy Loser clients told me. A year earlier, Sue and her sister-in-law both gave birth to healthy babies within a week of each other.

They walked their babies in their prams most mornings for an hour, and both new mums had gone back to work three months ago. But what got Sue's gander up was that she was still carrying an extra 10 kg after her baby's birth, and the skinny sister-in-law was 2 kg lighter than before she got pregnant. Frustrating? Sure is.

I asked Sue to tell me more about her sister-in-law's lifestyle and habits, as I already knew everything about Sue's energy-in, energy-out routine. Turns out the skinny sister-in-law had gone back to work nursing. She was an accident and emergency nurse, and ran her legs off for most of the eight hours she was on duty. I explained to Sue that after their hour walk in the morning, her sister-in-law clocked up another seven or eight hours of walking and, in some cases, running. There was no way Sue could match that, as she was an office worker with eight hours spent at a desk in front of a computer screen.

This is the root of many misconceptions about skinny people, slow metabolism, big bones, or the latest fat excuse: The new fat gene. All output is output, and being on your feet at work is going to burn a lot more calories than sitting behind a desk.

You don't have to take my word for it. There is a table of calculations called the METs Table, with a MET score for all activities we do.

MET refers to "Metabolic Equivalent of a Task", and is a reading of calories burned per hour, per kilo of weight. Sitting is ranked at 1 MET; therefore, if you weigh 65 kilos and sit for an hour, you've burned 65 calories. Every task you do has a MET reading; below is a brief breakdown:

- **Sitting or sleeping:** 1 and under.

- **Light activities, like casual walking or desk work:** 3 and under.

- **Moderate activities,** like cycling under 15 km an hour, light housework, and jobs that require being on your feet like teaching and retail: 4 and under.

- **Vigorous activities,** like running, fast cycling, race walking, and active jobs such as construction work or nursing: 5 or more depending on how active the job or activity is.

The MET reading shows that the heavier we are, the more calories we burn off per activity because it takes more exertion to move the bulk around. Therefore, if you weigh 100 kg, you burn off 100 calories sitting and up to 300 calories easy walking per hour. The example above of Sue and her skinny sister-in-law, could mean a difference of 1000 calories or more over their eight hour work day.

What does all this mean for Sue? Should she accept that she will always be the fat sister-in-law? Should she change jobs?

The most important thing for Sue is to stop comparing herself to her skinny sister-in-law. Sue loves her job, and would hate to have her sister-in-law's job, so she needs to set her own rules for her lifestyle. She may need to exercise more when she is not at work or cut back on some calories, or look at any bad eating habits she has (for example, often desk jobs create an easy-snacking environment).

Overheard in a podiatrist's office: "The wear pattern on your running shoes suggests you watch too much TV."

The moral of the "Skinny Sister-in-Law" story is to stop comparing yourself and your weight to everyone else. After creating Lazy Loser and fitness programs for years, I've never had one person's diet and exercise routine, work, and lifestyle be the same.

What we eat, how much we eat, and how we exercise is minimal in the scheme of our daily activities. Think about it: There are 24 hours in a day, and we're spending maybe two hours eating and exercising deliberately. That leaves 22 hours! What are we doing in that time? Yes, sleeping plays into it — I sleep five to six hours a night; others I know sleep eight to 10 hours.

But how much time are we sitting? And not just for work, but in cars, in front of the TV, at the computer, etc.? What we're doing in those 14 extra hours is likely to be contributing greatly to our weight gain. All the hours outside the two in which we're eating and deliberately exercising and the five to 10 during which we're sleeping are made up of incidental exercise. This is proven to play a big role in how fat we are, and how efficiently we burn calories.

Here are a few examples of incidental exercise:

- Walking to the shop
- Shopping
- Taking the stairs not the elevator
- Playing footy, hide and seek or chasey with the kids
- Getting up to change TV channels
- Cycling to work
- Gardening
- Housework
- Walking the dog
- Fidgeting!

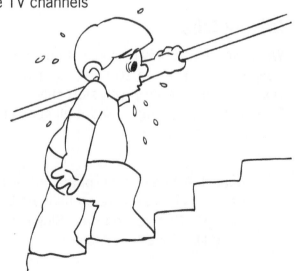

This is only the tip of the iceberg; you could probably think of lots more. But in a nutshell, it's getting up and doing something — anything. The invention of the remote control has taken a major incidental move away from us. Two-car families means we all drive. The death of the corner shop for the paper, bread, and milk takes away the early morning walk. We probably didn't even realise how much we were moving back then, but added up, these small moves made a big difference. We're still eating the same (more, in fact), but we don't move the way we used to. And it all adds up to fat.

Go back to your Lazy Loser scales. Is the input side making a dent in the counter while the output side floats in thin air?

What is the answer? No, you don't have to run on the treadmill for two hours instead of one, and you don't have to starve yourself (in fact, please don't). But if you like food like I do, then look at the output. Could you be out and about on your feet more?

Desk Jobs

You're not chained to that desk. Maybe you feel like you are, but physically, you're not.

There is an epidemic of people who now eat lunch at their desks in front of their computers. Don't do that. On each break, get up and move. Don't go from your desk to the tea room and sit again. Stand, walk around, or even leave the workplace — take your lunch to the park, and eat it there.

Driving Jobs

When you stop for any reason, get out of your car, bus, or truck and walk around for five to 10 minutes. If you stop a lot, that's lots of walks. However, even if you stop only three times, that's an extra 30 minutes of walking — and it all goes into the right side of your Lazy Loser scales.

Although Australia is one of the fattest nations, Bloomberg rates it at number three on their world-healthiest-country rankings. Number one is Singapore, two Italy, four Switzerland, and fifth Japan.

And as we discussed in Chapter 2, make it a habit, not a thought or an idea. It's something you do each time you have a break: You stand and walk.

Add up how much energy you could use riding your bike to work, or walking to the bus stop two blocks away. Double it for the homeward journey. Does that bring the output scale out of the clouds a bit?

On-your-feet jobs

These people should be skinny minis, right? Well, we know that's not the case, as many people in active jobs struggle with their weight as well. The active workers are often feeling physically exhausted at the end of their shifts, and the last thing they want to do is head to the gym or go for a run.

But that doesn't mean that going home, sitting on the couch and eating and drinking all night is the way to go, either. The amount of food and drink we consume is the biggest reason for weight gain, regardless of how active we are, and the left side of your Lazy Loser scales always needs to be looked at if you want to lose weight.

If you have a very active job and you are overweight, you need to look at the food side and halve the yummy stuff you're eating — yes, literally cut it down the middle. Share the other half with someone, or wrap it in cling wrap and eat it tomorrow. Don't like that idea? I see mini muffins now — what a great idea. There are lots of mini versions of food around – get on it!

Lazy Bottom Line

• It's your weight and health that are the issues, not other peoples. Be selfish: It's all about you.

• Stop comparing yourself to others; there will always be people thinner and fatter than you, get used to it. Don't spend energy (and that is the energy that doesn't burn calories) wondering why or worrying about how they stay thin. You cannot walk a mile in their shoes, so you'll never know how they do it. Walk miles in your own shoes.

• Incidental exercise is a major factor in weight gain and loss. The energy used in sitting, lying down, standing, and walking is very different. All of these things are easy to do and will not exhaust you, but some (standing and walking) will burn more calories than others (sitting and lying down). This is a simple way to add energy to the right side of your Lazy Loser scales.

• Adjust your lifestyle. If you sit at work all day, walk or cycle to and from work to counteract the sitting. If you have a sit-down job, accept that you will not burn as many calories as people who work in active jobs and you may need to eat less on working days. If you're active on the weekend, you can afford to eat more.

• Just because you're in an active job doesn't give you license to eat anything and everything. If you're eating and drinking too much, you will get fat.

Pacific-island nations have the highest average BMI in the world, reaching 34 to 35 kg/m^2 — up to 70% higher than some countries in Southeast Asia and sub-Saharan Africa. Among high-income countries, the U.S. has the highest BMI (over 28 kg/m^2 for men and women), followed by New Zealand. Japan has the lowest BMI (about 22 kg/m^2 for women and 24 kg/m^2 for men), followed by Singapore.

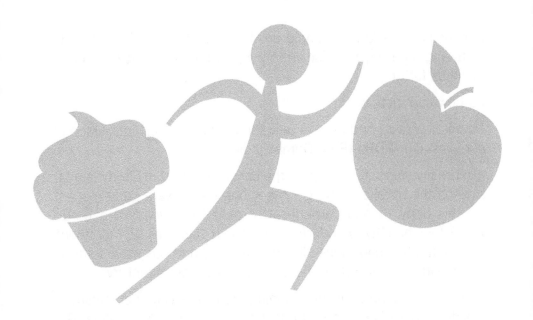

Chapter 7 – The Elephant in the Room: Diet

This chapter is not about comparing all the weird and wonderful diets out there. Let's assume we've heard of or tried many of them, and most people who have tried them are still overweight or struggling with their weight, and leave it at that.

I, like many, have dieted, although my dieting days were a while ago. I followed the ones in women's magazines or diets I heard about through word of mouth from all my dieting buddies. I didn't have the internet then; thank goodness, as I'd still be trying the "Get the body you want in 10 days!" diet 7,568 days later!

Numerous studies worldwide have yielded the same results: Diets don't work in the long term. A comprehensive study in the U.S. found that after people tried a weight-loss program, one-third to two-thirds of the weight was regained within a year. Another study found that most diets fail before the goal weight is reached, and in the long term, dieters became fatter after ending the diet.

The consensus is that most people on diets feel hungry and are even more preoccupied with food while on the diet. We all have a hormone called ghrelin; it's the one that makes us hungry, and its production increases by 20% when we're on a diet. However, the good hormones we have that supress hunger and stimulate metabolism are low in people on diets. It's like our body rejects diets and as a payback for attempting to go on one, it decides to make us fatter.

So how can diets work?

I think now is a good time to talk about a very important person in our lives: Our PDBs (Poor Dumb Bodies).

After many years, I've come to the conclusion that my body is a bit slow on the uptake. Don't get me wrong — I have a great respect for this body. It has carried and expelled (for want of a better word) four healthy, wonderful children. It has run 12 marathons and even ultra-marathons all over the world and has stayed strong and healthy, never letting me down for over half a century.

Sure, it has done a bit of whinging along the way, but mostly it has done what I've asked it to do without too much grumbling. But to be honest, if it had its way, PDB would be sitting in its cave, scratching its head and bum, and venturing out only once in a while with its club to chase down some poor dumber animal, just like its ancestors.

This is true for all of our PDB. We may think we've evolved a long way from our cave-dwelling days, but left to its own devices, PDB would be back there in a second.

You may have goals, dreams, and aspirations for your body shape and size, but PDB has only one goal for you: Survival. And if you're reading this right now, so far it's doing its job. Every waking moment, PDB is working for this great cause, and even when you're asleep it still has one eye on the ball.

Our bodies will go to any length to keep us alive. Think about it: One tiny, unseen-by-the-naked-eye germ finds its way into us via food, and PDB will continually expel and explode until it's been truly removed. One silly move by you with a knife, and PDB doesn't just bleed out — it activates coagulation and starts to close the wound immediately, saving your life.

South Korea, Cambodia, Australia, Canada, and the U.S. had some of the lowest blood pressures for both men and women: below 120 mmHg for women and 125 mmHg for men.

PDB and diets

The only problem is that PDB can be a bit slow to catch on in some areas. It has so much going on inside to keep it occupied that when you start on your beaut diet, the new eating plan slips under the radar for a bit. Your no-carb, low-fat diet starts with a bang. You begin dropping kilos in only a week, love your scales, and think, This is it: Skinny jeans, here I come!

However, after a couple of weeks, PDB starts to twig: *Where's my energy? My pretty fat stores that I've lovingly nurtured over years are starting to desert me! Hang on a minute . . . I'm starving, I'm going to die!* That's when PDB pulls the big red alarm cord; everything inside you stops and goes into damage control.

PDB doesn't see that you only want to shed a few extra kilos that you don't need. It is in for the long term, it thinks you've run out of food, and is looking after you by holding onto energy and fat stores until you can get out of the cave and find more. That's when the scales stop being your best friend. When you're eating under 1,000 calories a day and nothing is happening, you get frustrated and angry and eat the biggest chocolate muffin you can find. PDB is happy, because once again it has saved your life!

Scientists and the mega junk-food industry have tried to trick PDB over the years with wonderful new inventions designed to make you feel full or taste sweetness without the actual sugar fix. And yes, PDB goes along for some of the ride, but when it wakes up and discovers it has been duped, it fights back. The end result is that we're fatter, and PDB is victorious again.

Diet drinks are a classic example: Zero calories, but sweet and they taste the same as the real stuff. What a great invention. If you used to drink the sugared variety by the gallon but swap to the zero-sugar kind and drank two gallons, you should lose weight, and all soft-drink addicts will now be skinny.

The trouble is the intended result hasn't happened. People who drink low or zero-calorie soft drinks have reported no weight loss, and in fact, many have gained weight. How can that be? They've taken a big chunk of empty calories out of their diet.

Once again, blame PDB. When you drink or eat something with a sugar substitute, PDB thinks "I love this stuff! It makes me feel good and gives me lots of energy to complete my mission, which is to keep this idiot alive." However, as PDB isn't so quick on the uptake, it enjoys the taste and the sensation the fake sugar gives to the brain, but after a while the penny drops:

"Hey, wait a minute . . . where's all my energy from the sugar? It's not working; I've been ripped off!"

It then sets off a chant to the brain: "We want sugar! We want the real stuff! We want sugar!", so off you go to buy a block of chocolate, restoring the balance. Yes, fake sugar is okay for taste — but the body only works on the real thing.

Sweet things make you crave sweet things; fake sweet things make you crave real sweet things. That's PDB law.

Over the years, I've tried to listen to PDB, and I know this is what it would tell us if it could talk:

1. I'm the ultimate hoarder; overeat, and I'm hanging onto that fat for a rainy day.

2. I can smell a rat! Don't try to trick me with your good-tasting, low-fat foods; they don't satisfy my organs and systems, and I'll demand more of the real thing.

3. Drink all the grog you want tonight, but I'm going to make you suffer for at least 24 hours while I try getting it through your liver and kidneys; these things take time.

4. Vitamin and mineral supplements? I see — trying to trick me again. I'll let the kidney and bladder deal with them, and out they go.

5. Don't go cold turkey on anything, because I won't be happy, I need to be weaned.

Cold showers for another reason! A blast of cold water at the end of your shower is said to renew energy levels. The stimulation of the chilly water to the sympathetic nervous system causes our brains to produce adrenaline.

6. I need fat, protein, carbs, vitamins, and minerals to function. I don't care how you get them to me, but I have to have them in the right amounts. Not enough of each and I won't do what you want me to do.

7. I'm not interested in how you look on the outside, but I'd prefer you at the right weight, as it makes it easier for me to move around and get things done. I can store all your excess fat, but it gives me more work to do, so I'm never going to be as efficient as I could be if you were the right weight.

Be nicer to PDB

We're very tough on PDB. Not only do we want it to keep us alive, but it has to look and feel stunning and gorgeous 100% of the time. When we check it in the mirror and don't like what we see, boy is it in for some trouble.

PDB deals with the 'energy-in' side and processes the food and drink we consume; however, it's a bit different for the 'energy-out' side, and this is where the mind takes charge.

PDB will do anything you ask of it, physically; it just goes along for the ride. Sure it whinges or moans a bit, but basically it follows you around all day every day doing what you ask. It's in this area that you can control PDB and, in turn, your health and weight.

Lazy Tale

Loser Tales are snippets of events and opinions that have resonated with me over the years in regard to food, fat, and fitness. Often, I think I've heard and seen it all — and then something comes along that shocks or surprises me, which is great. An occasion like this happened while I was writing this book.

I wrote half of "Lazy Loser" in London. I was there to launch my first publication, "Lazy Runner", and also holding book talks and running workshops. During one workshop in Victoria Park, I was told that there was to be a bike ride in London that afternoon, with an extra twist:

All the cyclists would be nude! It was the annual nude World Naked Bike Ride to promote safe cycling in the city.

That sounds like fun! I thought, so off to Waterloo Bridge I went to wait with my camera at the ready; I'm not prude when it comes to nude! I was a nurse for 20 years so I saw the odd bod, but full-on outdoor nudity was something I'd never encountered.

And let me tell you — WOW! There were thousands of butt-naked cyclists. Some had discreet body paint and delicately placed flowers and G-strings here and there, but the majority were stripped down to their birthday suits.

I learned two things that day. One was that there is no perfect body. The bikers were not ugly, gross, sexy, or stunning — they were just all different. Each cyclist had all their bits and pieces in the right place, but that is where the similarity ended. Most had boobs (yes, some of the fellas too): Big, little, saggy. They also had bums: Big, little, saggy. And each had a belly: Big, little, saggy. Do I need to go on?

The nude cyclists were a good cross section of society: Tall, short, old, young, different races, thin, curvy, etc. Not one of them had the bodies I'd seen naked and half naked in magazines or on billboards or TV. Which lead me to think, *Maybe those bodies are fake.* The bodies on Waterloo bridge were real; I can vouch that as an eyewitness. If the bodies we see on films, TV shows, and billboards are normal, then why didn't I see one on the nudie bike ride? Then it struck me: Those bodies in the media are not normal.

I think of all the people I've talked with over years about their weight, and how they're looking for their perfect body. I now know that that body has been conjured up from an image they have in their minds —a fictional one they saw in picture on a screen. I wish I could take all my clients onto Waterloo Bridge each year and say, "Okay, now have a look at this lot and pick your perfect body; it has to be one of these, as they are real bodies."

I said I learned two things that day. The other was not to use zoom on your camera when a large nude man gets a puncture on his bike and quickly jumps off and bends over to fix it. The camera didn't break, but the image was burned onto my retina for quite some time afterward!

How to trick your PDB

The way I've got my PDB to do what I want over the years is by sneaking up on it! The way to do this is to introduce something new discreetly, before PDB has twigged.

For instance, with running, I always say up your distance 10%, or half a kilometre, per week. You may run 5 km one day and think, Yay I'm good at this; I'm going to do 10 km tomorrow! Off you go and your body is behaving nicely. You get to 5 km and PDB says, "Been here, done this!" At 5.5 km, PDB is still not sure what's going on, but is happy to stick with it. You get to 7 km and PDB says, "Hey, wait a minute — I never signed up for this!" At 8 km, it's, "Blow this for a joke; I'm shutting up shop!" And then, of course, it's a sad, slow walk home.

You had it at 5.5 km; leave it there. Next time you will get PDB to 6 km before it twigs, and so on. This is how I've run marathons and ultra-marathons! If I push my body too hard, often it will do what I ask, but the pain and maybe even injury is never worth it.

It's the same with food intake; don't do anything cold turkey. You may know you eat too much sugar, but don't cut it all out. Take baby steps: Start with removing 1 tsp. from your tea and coffee. PDB is looking for its sugar fix, and it still gets that, keeping it happy.

The next week, take out some sugared drinks, like juice or soft drinks. Once your body has come to terms with that, take out a bit more. Before the body knows it (and it could take a month), you've halved your added-sugar consumption, and PDB is oblivious. The same goes for all your extra calories, alcohol, fatty foods, snack foods, etc. Baby steps.

Lazy Bottom Line

• Diets don't work. The majority of people gain back the lost weight and even more after finishing a diet.

• You know it's a diet if it has a timeframe; tells you how many kilos you'll lose and how long it will take; requires you to buy and eat pre-prepared meals or shakes; drastically cuts out certain food groups, advises you to take a multivitamin supplement, or you know you couldn't last on it for six months or more.

• Our bodies are designed to keep us alive; being overweight or eating poorly makes that job much harder for them.

• Your body will do whatever you tell it to do; it just goes along for the ride, so make sure you're telling it the right things.

• Be nice to your body, and stop fighting it; if you want to stay alive, let it do its job. If you'd like to change a few things about it, then be subtle; it will hardly notice and then, when it does, too late — the changes have been made and adapted. You win!

Western European countries like Greenland, Iceland, Andorra, and Germany have the highest cholesterol levels in the world, with mean serum total cholesterols of around 5.5 mmol/L. African countries have the lowest cholesterol — some as low as 4 mmol/L.

Chapter 8 – Rules

I like to watch the weight-loss reality shows on TV. I'm constantly amazed at the size of the contestants. These people are morbidly obese, unhappy about it, and wanting to change. The first question that comes into my head is, *How could it ever have got to that point? Why didn't they do something about it sooner?*

I wonder what their thought processes were when they reached 100 kg, 120 kg, 150 kg, and even 200 kg. How does this happen? I mean, I know how it happens: They're eating and drinking too much and not moving enough, but how can it go on and on without them putting the brakes on the out-of-control eating machine? I'd think XXL clothes being too tight would be a trigger. Maybe having to get a special seatbelt fitted in your car is a sign. What about when you can't fit in an airline seat?

Many of the morbidly obese contestants say their doctors have nearly given them their last rites, but they still couldn't stop overeating. At the start of the show, the new participants are filmed at home, and we get to see their eating patterns and lifestyles prior to entering the competition. We get a glimpse of their past lives before entering their new world of diet, deprivation, and continual butt-kicking.

We view in horror as they chow down on several meat pies in one sitting, eat a family-size pizza washed down with a litre of soft drink, or eating ice cream out of a two-litre tub as if it's a bowl. It's extreme overeating.

I chalk it up to having no rules when it comes to eating and exercising.

They wake up every day and do whatever they like. They eat and drink what's in front of them or in their fridges or pantries. When they eat out, they order whatever they want. When in the supermarket, anything and everything goes into the trolley. If they're not on a diet or eating plan, it's open slather on food and drink.

We all need rules in our lives. I'm not overweight, yet I have food and exercise rules I stick to. And I figure after years of having these rules, they're probably the reason I'm not overweight. They're not strict, crazy rules, but just a few guidelines that remind me to stay on track with my eating and health.

I've mentioned before that I love food — all food. To me, none is off bounds, and I really will have a go at anything. This is especially why I need to have a few rules; if I didn't, you'd see me getting my butt kicked on national TV.

I try not to eat randomly. By that, I mean I'll assess most things I eat and ask myself whether I need that right now, if it's the best choice, or if it's too much food for one person. And don't worry — there are many times I say to myself, "I don't need that right now, it's not the best choice, and it's too much . . . but who cares. I'm going to eat it anyway!" Luckily, that doesn't occur too often. This is known as a breach of the rules. And the punishment for my rule break? Go for a run!

I'm not obsessed with my rules, and often I don't even think about them until I'm faced with one of their temptations. It's a tiny warning bell that sits in the back of my consciousness, and if I break a rule, it gives me a little signal, saying something like, "Hey, what's going on? You just broke one of your rules!" Oops . . . sorry about that!

The 21st century sees us living undisciplined lives. When we want to quit something, we quit. When we want a new thing, we buy it (even if we don't have the money). Rules: What are they? Unless it's legally binding, we have no problem cheating or breaking promises; no, not all of us and not all the time, but it seems we find it easy to do in modern day society.

I think about my parents' and grandparents' lives. If there was food in the house, they'd never re-shop or throw it out; no more food would be bought until current stocks were depleted. They used cash to buy things, and if they didn't have the money, they went without.

Discipline is very important when it comes to ensuring we have a healthy life. Temptation is rampant; everywhere we look there is something yummy to eat, and we never have to go far to get that yummy thing. However, if you have a few simple rules in your life where food and exercise are concerned and you stick to those rules the majority of the time, it won't be long until you find you lose weight and get healthier without ever having to diet again.

I challenge you to pick three food-and-fitness rules from the list below and incorporate them into your daily lifestyle:

The rules

1. Don't eat while driving (this is one of mine).

2. Always opt for skim whenever having milk or yoghurt.

3. Only eat out once a week, this includes fast food.

4. Don't eat at the movies.

5. Don't eat while watching TV.

6. Exercise every day.

7. All exercise sessions must last at least 45 minutes.

8. Never have seconds after dinner, even if there are leftovers.

9. Don't eat sweets after dinner.

10. Only have one treat a day.

11. Drink alcohol only when you're out (never at home).

12. Eat five vegetable and two fruit servings per day.

13. Never eat out of a packet; put the food on a plate or bowl.

14. Always have breakfast.

15. Don't keep fizzy drinks in your fridge.

16. Don't add sugar from the bowl to anything cooked.

17. Don't add salt to anything cooked.

18. Don't eat after 8 p.m.

19. Take 10,000 steps a day (you'll need a pedometer).

20. Get up after each meal and move around for 15 to 30 minutes.

21. Never go more than 48 hours without having exercised.

22. Don't drive (or be a passenger in a car) anywhere unless it's more than three km from your home; all short trips must be done on foot or bike.

23. Stop eating when you're full.

24. Only eat on five or fewer separate occasions during the day; no eating in between.

25. Never take a lift (elevator) up or down five or fewer floors.

26. Move every hour during the day.

27. Never purchase food from a drive-thru.

28. Don't upsize meals.

29. Drink six to eight glasses of water a day.

30. Have only one coffee a day.

31. Don't eat in bed.

32. Don't eat in the middle of the night.

33. Have at least three alcohol free days a week.

34. Don't eat lollies.

35. Don't buy food or drink at petrol stations.

36. Never buy meals prefixed with super, whopper, double, or triple.

37. Cook only with olive oil.

38. Never eat anything deep fried.

39. Don't eat anything coated in crumbs or batter.

40. Don't add butter or margarine to anything on your plate.

41. Don't eat anything sweet for breakfast.

42. Buy more fresh, unpackaged food than packaged products weekly.

43. Cut all the food on your dinner plate by one quarter.

44. Brush your teeth directly after dinner and don't eat or drink again.

45. Ride your exercise bike or walk on a treadmill while you watch the evening news.

46. Only ever have a piece of fresh fruit (no other foods) between your three meals a day.

47. Never drink juices, flavoured waters, or bottled iced teas.

48. Never upsize a meal, no matter how cheap it is; always go for small or medium.

49. Never order fries or hot chips with your takeaways.

50. Don't have a sugar bowl in your house.

51. Don't have table salt in your house.

52. Exercise five mornings a week.

53. Walk the dog every day.

54. Have four processed-food-free days a week.

55. Cook five healthy dinners a week.

56. Have three meat-free dinners a week.

57. Don't have bread with your evening meal.

58. Always choose wholegrain breads and rolls.

59. Don't add creamy sauces to home cooked meals.

60. Cut TV/computer time/electronic games by half.

61. Eat slowly

Those are a lot of rules and you may even have some more to add; feel free to make up your own!

There are rules about the rules!

Straight away I can hear you thinking, "This is easy; I'll pick a rule that I never break anyway." I didn't come down in the last storm, I'm onto you lot! If you're a teetotaller, don't think I'm going to let you pick rule 11.

Similarly:

• If you hate fizzy drinks, you can't pick rule 15.

• If there are no drive-thru food outlets in your town, you can't pick rule 27.

• If you haven't encountered an elevator in the past week, you can't pick rule 25.

On the other hand:

• If you normally have three cappuccinos a day with two sugars in each, rule 30 is perfect for you.

• If you drink alcohol every day, go for rule 33.

• If you graze after dinner, rule 18 is yours.

Here's the deal...

If what you're doing now is causing you to gain or not lose weight, then nothing is going to change if you pick rules you're already good with. Your rules need to be about things you like doing but feel could make a difference if you stopped.

Japan has seen its average cholesterol in men and women rise from a low starting point in 1980 to the levels seen in the western world in 2008. Singapore saw cholesterol drop from 1980 to 2000, then rise substantially. China also saw increases in cholesterol, though its figures remain low in global terms. The patterns in Japan, China, and Singapore are likely to be at least partly due to changes in diet, including increasing intake of animal products and fats.

Once again, it's going back to habits — this time, the good ones. You pick three rules and make them part of your daily life. It could take a few weeks to adapt to them or even remember them. But after a month or so, they become habit and part of who you are and what you do.

You'll plan out the best time to have that one coffee; walk past the elevator and not even think about it; when you put your sports shoes on you will know that you have to be exercising for 45 minutes. When this happens, you're set; weight loss will come your way just from these three new habits you made for yourself.

Like figures? Here are some for you:

Rule 3: Drop 14 kg a year by skipping two fast food meals (1,200 calories [Big Mac Meal] plus 850 calories [foot-long meatball Subway sub and diet drink] = 2050 calories a week X 52 weeks / 7,700 [calories in 1 kg]).

Rule 20: If the movement is walking, you'll burn 6 kg per year (125 calories [15 minutes X 3 meals] X 365 days / 7,700).

Rule 30: Dropping from three skim cappuccinos with two sugars to one per day equals a loss of 13 kg a year (140 calories X 2 x 365 days / 7,700).

So if your rules are 3, 20, and 30 and you keep all other food and activity the same, you could lose 33 kg a year! Even if you allow for a few rule breaks here and there and stuck to the rules 75% of the time, that's still nearly 25 kg a year. That's amazing!

Maybe you're not as strict with your rules as you could be and stick to them 50% of the time, but that's still 16.5 kg. You have to be happy with those figures compared to the minimal effort you've put in. No diet or boot camp in sight – just three new life rules.

Work it out for yourself: Pick your three rules and calculate what difference the rules are going to make. If it's energy, find out how many calories you'll burn from implementing your rule. If it's food, look at how many calories you're likely to reduce daily or weekly from the change. Get it to a yearly calorie figure, then divide by 7,700 calories, and the answer is the kilos you can expect to lose in a year from your three rules.

Rule 1	Rule 2	Rule 3
ECC=-	ECC=-	ECC=-
X 365 days OR 52 weeks =	X 365 days OR 52 weeks =	X 365 days OR 52 weeks =
ACS =	ACS =	ACS =
÷7700	÷7700	÷7700
= kilos lost per year:	= kilos lost per year:	= kilos lost per year:

ECC = Expected Calorie Change; ACS = Annual Calories Saved

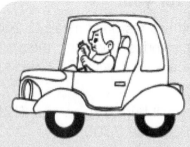

Lazy Tale

My rules have changed over the years, as my lifestyle and food tastes have altered. I've been known to occasionally buy some snacks from the lovely lady who upsells the goodies where I buy petrol. Then back in the car 10 km up the road, the bag of jelly snakes is gone. Who ate them? I don't know. I remember having about three or four (okay, maybe five or six), but there's no way I ate the lot.

When I had young children it was okay — I could blame them — but now I have to face the harsh reality that I ate a whole bag of jelly snakes! This type of behaviour didn't happen very often, as I lived and worked in one place for seven years; my travelling was to running coaching sessions between 4 and 5 a.m. Even someone with a sweet tooth like me had trouble facing those little red snakes at that time of day. So a rule wasn't necessary.

Last year, I wrote my first book "Lazy Runner" and hit the road on a book-and-running workshop tour across Australia. It's a big country, so lots of driving. I stopped at a service station once or twice a day, and no matter where in the country I was, there was always a lovely attendant trying to upsell me lollies with my petrol.

I had to make a new rule: No buying food at the service station, and another one: No eating in the car. It was tough on both counts. I craved the company of my little snakes on the long, lonely road, but if I wanted something to eat and drink, I had to get out of the car to do it. Sometimes I found that frustrating, as I just wanted to keep driving; however, stopping each time to eat made me walk around and stretch my legs, which helped. So for four months my rules were 1, 20, and 35.

On the four-month trip, I probably broke my rules five times. But that was okay with me, as if I didn't have the rules, I'd have eaten a million lolly snakes over the 10,000 kms (6000 miles)!

The moral of this Loser Tale is to set the rules that are relevant to you right now. Your rules should relate to something that affects you on a daily basis, or several times a week. If things change in your life and your rules become obsolete, pick new ones.

I don't need exercise or activity rules, as that part of my lifestyle is easy. I like to exercise; it's my habit, and I miss it if I can't do it. Food is my Achilles heel; therefore, all my rules usually revolve around sweets, overeating, and alcohol consumption.

Lazy Bottom Line

• Obesity mostly comes from eating whatever you like and being as lazy as you want to be.

• Set a few simple food and exercise rules for yourself; getting them to the point where they are habit can be enough to make you lose kilos annually.

• Your rules should be relevant to unhealthy habits you may have developed over the years.

• Choose your rules based on things you do daily or several days a week.

- Throw out a rule whenever it no longer fits in with your lifestyle, and pick another one to replace it.

- It's fine to be naughty and break the rules every so often, but aim to stick to them 75% of the time.

- Don't choose a rule you know you can't follow; you'll fail at sticking to it and get disappointed. For instance, if you hate the taste of tea without sugar, that's okay — pick a rule you can get your head around and stick to it. It's no good setting a rule you break daily.

- If you break a rule continually (more than 50% of the time), change it to another rule; if it's not working for you, it's not worthwhile to keep persisting with it.

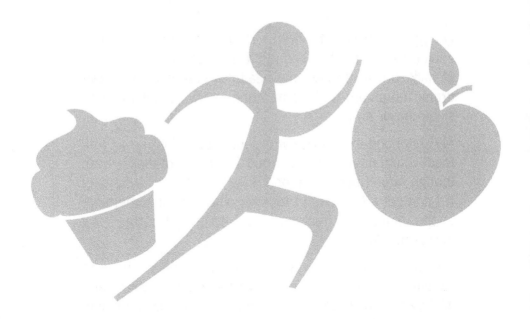

Chapter 9 – Not Fat-Free...Free Fat

Lazy Tale

Do you remember the free-milk programs at school? This was when the Milkos would dump a few crates of little bottles of full-cream milk in the school playgrounds. They would sit in the sun for two hours, and at playtime we were all marched out and had to drink a bottle of warm milk.

Boy, I hated that milk. I would nearly gag when the shiny little foil lid came off, and on top of the milk would be a thick yellow layer of hot cream.

Some kids would get out of having to drink the milk, because their mums would write a letter to the school with an excuse about lactose intolerance or some such thing. I would beg mum to get me out of the school milk program, but her answer was always, "It's free and you will drink it, and what's more, you will bloody well like it!" Mum used to add that last bit to most sentences when we would whinge about anything — washing dishes, going to church, getting a clip across the ear, etc.

For years I obeyed the first part of mum's demand, but I couldn't abide by the second bit. I am still not a great fan of milk, but it did help my health in one way: I've never drunk full-cream milk as an adult; I always opt for semi skimmed or no fat.

My childhood experience with food instilled in me a "free food" mentality, and I'm afraid it's hard to shake; even though I don't need free food now, I can't resist a freebie! If I can get a free bite of food, or a sample of something, to the ultimate in freebies — a free cup of coffee — it makes my day.

I've also learned to latch onto the free nibbles in supermarkets. I've chowed down on cereal, muesli bars, all types of new beverages, and even kebabs and rice. One day whilst grocery shopping I was so full I wondered if I should just ditch the trolley and go home, then come back later and see what was on the menu for dinner!

I like food deals; I'm hooked on two-for-ones and pay-for-one-and-get-another-half-price deals. But it does lead me to wonder how much extra I eat just because I got it free. Personally, I think all free food should be calorie free; if you're not paying for it with your wallet, why should your hips suffer?

The basics of Lazy Loser are to watch how much we eat and eat healthier when possible. But there are plenty of temptations out there, and it's easy to fall victim to them. Even if you're strictly following a low-sugar rule with your diet, it's very hard to pass up a free chocolate offered to you by a very friendly, smiling lady, and then maybe just one more of a different flavour. Or, what the hell — might as well buy the block because she was so nice. Wait, two blocks for the price of one? Well, it's just silly not to take that offer, I mean, someone will eat it! Unfortunately that someone is most likely to be you.

More is cheaper in our society; buy-one-get-one-free deals are rampant, the bigger size is as cheap as the smaller one, etc. And where does all the free, bigger stuff end up? Inside "someone".

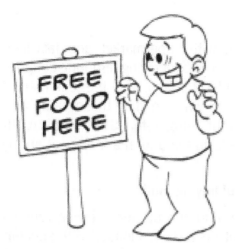

One rule I made for myself once (see Chapter 8: Rules) was to have no free food, no two-for-ones, and no upsizing for a month. It was hard — everywhere I went, deals were jumping out at me, or nice ladies in supermarkets were chasing me with trays full of yummy treats to try.

That wasn't the case, of course, but that's how it felt. I decided to remove myself from the supermarket temptation scene for a while and buy my food at farmers' markets. But that was worse — they have free samples everywhere! They were healthy, but as we know, not always low in calories — especially the delicious Greek yoghurt samples.

Think all those little samples mean nothing for your weight? Well, it's all calories, and it adds up. Every time you buy a two-for-one or upsized product, you drink and eat more of it; maybe not immediately, but over time. Remember: If it's not there, you can't eat it. Usually it's the multinational food companies that offer amazing two-for-one deals on the junky types of food like lollies, chocolates, fizzy drinks, and chips. Very rarely do you see two-for-one deals on healthy products like fruits and veggies.

Here are some tips on how to not fall into freebie or upsize traps:

1. Cut your ties with the supermarket.

Don't go daily or even weekly to the supermarket; do a fortnightly or monthly shop. You may think you buy more, but you will eat less this way.

When you get home with your huge bundle of groceries, sort it into smaller, meal-sized portions. For example, divide up big packets of meat and freeze it into just enough for each member of the household's serving size per meal. This way you avoid all the weekly sales, or new deals that suck you in and make you buy more.

2. Ban the junk mail.

If your letterbox is overflowing with supermarket and fast-food catalogues, stop the junk mail. If you're receiving tempting coupons or offers for amazing meals and food prices, stop the junk mail. If you have your scissors next to you while reading these pamphlets or lots of coupons pinned to your refrigerator, STOP THE JUNK MAIL! What you don't know won't hurt you (or make you eat or buy more food).

3. Put someone else in charge of buying food.

Do you go into the supermarket and end up nearly giving yourself a hernia carrying the basket out because it's loaded with specials you had no intention of buying when you walked through the door? Then give yourself the sack.

There's probably someone else in your home who could take over the shopping reins — a partner, a teenager, a roommate, your poor old mum, anyone. Write down your shopping list, give it to them, and let them loose in the supermarket. Tell them only to buy the items on the list, and then you've removed all temptation. It will cost you less, as well.

4. Determine who the best shopper is.

Believe it or not, shopping, like many things, is a natural talent; some are good at it, and others are terrible.

If you have a partner or roommate, take turns shopping every week. After a couple of months, you'll soon learn who the best, healthiest, and most economical shopper is. Take note how much unhealthy food, wasted food, or whether too much food is brought into the house each week.

Often, mums are relegated to the shopping and cooking whether they have a talent for it or even like it. But maybe someone else in the house has a natural flair for cooking and food shopping. Life would be so much better if everyone did the job they were best at — even grocery shopping.

5. Make a list.

This is the easiest thing to do — the hardest part is sticking to it!

Look through your pantry and fridge, and only put things on the list you're going to run out of or need for meals over the next week or two. When you get to the supermarket, follow the list to the letter, and don't buy two of anything you don't need.

Before you get to the checkout, go through the trolley, remove things that are not on the list, and find a nice attendant who will go and put it all back. If you try this once and you can't stick to your list, or you get home with five or more things that weren't on the list, sack yourself and go back to Tip 3.

6. Shop online.

Who would have ever thought you could buy groceries while sitting at home in your pyjamas, and then get them delivered to your house? I'm not sure they put the food away for you yet, but I hope that service is coming.

Many of the people I know who do their grocery shopping online say there's no going back, as it's convenient, they only order what they need, and it's often cheaper and healthier since they get only what they order.

7. Stop using credit for food.

I raised four children before credit cards were the rage they are now. I had to take a certain amount of cash to the supermarket for my weekly shop, and there was many an embarrassing occasion when the end tally would be far more than the amount of money I had in my wallet. So of course, I had to put things back.

What did I put back? The things I came in and had no intention of buying, but were on sale or looked yummy. But now that we all have credit, when the final tally comes up we may be shocked, but we just hand over the plastic and off we go, with far more food than we need.

According to a 2008 study by the School of Public Health at Imperial College London, more than one in 10 of the world's adult population was obese, with women more likely to be obese than men. An estimated 205 million men and 297 million adult women were obese — a total of more than half a billion adults worldwide.

Go back to cash. Work out an estimate of how much money you need for the groceries, take that amount of money, and leave the credit card at home. When you go over your cash budget (and you invariably will), things will have to go back.

When you get to the checkout, put all the healthy foods on the belt first and all the unhealthy, sweet, or added extras last. Once your budget has been reached, that's it — whatever's left on the belt stays at the supermarket.

8. Beware a bargain.

Something is only a bargain if you need it and it's good for you. These rules never seem to apply to food bargains.

Upsizing on fast-food meals: Usually, the upsize is one-third more fries and fizzy drink. These are the part of the meal with empty calories; you don't need them, and they'll make you fat. That is not a bargain.

Two-for-one or buy-one-get-one-half-price deals: When you go to the supermarket, do you go with the intention of buying two blocks of chocolate, or two tubs of ice cream? I bet you never do, yet that is what you often go home with because you got a bargain. But what you're actually doing is taking unhealthier, sugar-laden food into your house. That is not what you need, is not good for you, and is therefore not a bargain.

Lazy Bottom Line

- Free food still has calories (sometimes more than the food you pay for).

- Buying two of a product can be cheaper, but you'll pay for it in the long run.

- Supermarkets are deadly to people who can't resist a bargain or a freebie. If you're in this group, stop doing the grocery shop.

Healthiness of the food we eat decreases by 1.7% for every hour that passes in the day.

Lazy Loser

- Always have a shopping list, and don't deviate from it.

- Take cash to the supermarket; leave the credit card at home.

- Put a "No Junk Mail" sign on your letterbox.

- Never upsize a meal, or buy a food bargain; neither is ever the healthy option.

On average, people who don't eat breakfast eat 6.8% more food throughout the day.

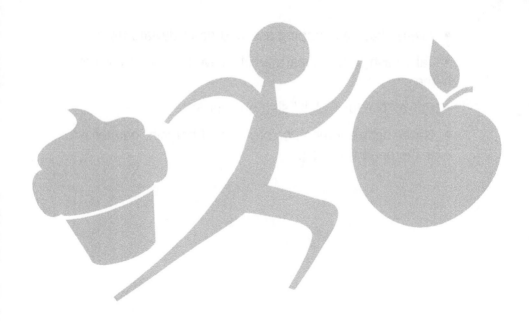

Chapter 10 – Don't Count or Read ... Just Look

I said at the beginning that this was not a diet book, so it doesn't follow the rules of your usual books on health, fitness, and eating.

I've read (maybe browsed is the better word) lots of diet and fitness books, and they all seem to contain the same layout:

- A few chapters on why we're fat and how to change that.
- Lots of colourful recipes for healthy meals and snacks.
- Pictures of thin people exercising.
- Charts, food-label explanations, and calorie counters.
- Pages and pages of diet plans for the reader to follow.

My problems with these books are:

- As a member of planet Earth for 50 years, I long ago figured out what makes me fat (food) and how to be not so fat (eat less). I'm sceptical when I read books espousing new scientific theories on food and weight loss.

- I follow the recipe section like a toddler, oohing and aaahhhing over the pretty pictures and wishing someone would prepare them for me, as I know if I did it myself, they'd never look or taste as good.

• I look at the exercises, but never feel motivated to do them on my own at home.

• I'm too lazy to chart and research everything that goes into my mouth, or follow a food plan.

The health/diet industry doesn't credit us with having a brain, and assumes we don't understand the concept of eating and exercising. You'd have had to live in a cave for the last 20 years with no TV, magazines, radio, or newspapers not to know that eating too much and not moving enough will make us fat. Telling it in a different way or finding a new fad for us to latch onto doesn't help, and only adds to the confusion — and in the meantime, the world gets fatter.

Many of the experts now tell us to watch what we eat by counting calories, reading food labels, and researching the food we eat. The thought of doing all that makes me tired (oh, and hungry as well!).

What is a calorie?

I mention calories a lot in this book — not in calorific allowances, but that each food has calories (some more than others). It's important to know that fact.

A calorie is a measurement of heat energy (well, that's the way the body measures calories). Heat is energy, and energy comes from food. The heat energy fuels our body; it comes into the body in many different forms and sources — some with lots of heat energy, and some not so much. Fats have the highest amount of heat energy at around 9 calories per gram, and carbohydrates and protein carry less at around 4 calories per gram. And, just for my benefit, I'll throw this one into the mix: Pure alcohol has about 7 calories per gram!

How many calories do we need to eat?

Here is another loaded question. We need to eat enough energy to stay alive, and if we eat too much, we have more energy than we know what to do with. So this extra energy sticks around: On our bums, bellies, and hips! And no, there's not a fine line in between — it's a huge, gaping chasm, with lots of yummy stuff in the middle.

Daily calorie allocations are based on the height, weight, age, and sex of a person. Men can eat more calories per day than women; they burn more heat energy than females, as they have more muscle mass and are usually bigger. Children and pregnant woman have different levels as well: Both generally require more heat energy to grow.

Very broad figures tell us that the average calorie consumption to maintain weight is 2,200 for women and 2,500 for men; however, this figure is based on a normal-activity lifestyle. People who are sporty or in active jobs burn more calories and therefore can consume more.

If you want to lose weight, you need to reduce the daily tally, and if you want to gain weight, you add to it. This is the basic answer, but do we need to know more? Sure, it fluctuates, and there are many other factors that come into play, but knowing how many calories we need in order to lose weight, stay the same, or put on weight would mean we'd have to know our exact daily total, and then count all the calories we eat to make sure we're in the right range. Which leads me to announce . . .

Counting calories is a bore!

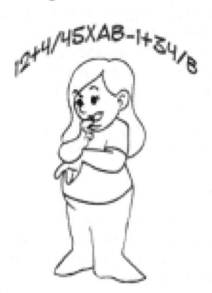

Yes, we know all foods have calories and that all are different, but do we really have to count all of them? I once looked up a calorie counter online to see how many calories were in an apple. There were over 25 choices of apple! I had to scroll through to find mine, and I still don't know if it was the right one. Was it peeled, stewed, cored,

Sunday is the unhealthiest eating day of the week.

canned, sliced, diced? Was it green, red, large, small? Was it in a pie? Did it have sugar on top? Going through them turned me into a crab-apple (which, by the way, I think had 18 calories, but I can't be totally sure!).

Knowing how many calories are in each food could easily be turned into a science degree that would never end: You'd have to keep getting post-graduate diplomas to keep up with the thousands of new food products that hit our supermarkets shelves annually, not to mention all the wonderful new recipes invented daily.

I say - don't even bother starting. If you have a life outside of eating and drinking — which I hope most of us do — then don't waste it on calorie counting.

Don't count — go with your gut (instinct, that is)

If your dinner is piled high on your plate or hanging over the sides, it means you have too many calories on there. If the food you're about to eat is dripping in oil or covered in sugar, it's dripping in calories as well. If you're eating something that was handed to you through the window of your car, you may be consuming half your daily calories in one go.

Remember: Food is not out to trick or con you — that's the food manufacturer's job. If your food is fresh and not packaged, you know it probably has fewer calories than food with writing all over it.

Daily Food Plan 1 Example:

Breakfast: If you eat wholegrain toast or two crumpets (even if they have some butter on them), or a healthy cereal or porridge; eggs on toast; fruit, or yoghurt for breakfast, you've probably consumed no more than 500 calories.

Lunch: You may eat a meat-and-salad roll or wrap; or a quiche; soup and roll; salad, or even a meat pie, but you've probably consumed no more than 600 to 700 calories.

Dinner: If you serve up the right serving size of steak, chicken, or fish with vegetables and potatoes, rice, or pasta, you'll probably eat no more than 600 to 800 calories.

You could even have some snacks in between: A couple of pieces of fruit, a chocolate biscuit, a mini muffin, a cup of yoghurt, etc. that could add on another 300 to 400 calories.

That's a lot of food, and it's still under or close to the magic 2,000 to 2,500 calories.

Daily Food Plan 2 Example:

Breakfast: The works: two fried eggs, bacon, sausage, baked beans, toast with butter, coffee, and juice could end up being more than 900 calories.

Lunch: Pie, chips, and a can of Coke: approximately 900 calories.

Dinner: Chicken Kiev, scalloped potatoes, steamed veggies, two slices of garlic bread, and two glasses of wine: over 1000 calories.

Add in a couple of snacks in between and you're over 3,000. As you can see, Plan 2 has lots of food as well, but a lot more calories.

The difference between the two plans

If you eat most of the types of foods on the first daily list, you should stay the same weight and, depending on your activity levels, you could lose weight over a year.

If you partake in the foods and drinks on the second plan and continue to do that for a year, it would add up to an extra 3,500 calories a week. It's estimated there are 7,700 calories in a kilo. That means you could easily gain a kilo a fortnight on that diet, which could put on over 30 kg in one year.

However, I suggest eating a selection from both lists. Sometimes, we eat too much or pig out on greasy food and takeaways, and at other times, we eat well and healthy. Maybe you start the day with a healthy bowl of porridge with skim milk, but at lunch you can't go without your meat pie. You may eat the chicken Kiev and garlic bread at the pub once a week for dinner, but on the other nights, you cook a healthy dinner for yourself.

On average, dinner is 15.9% unhealthier than breakfast.

The trick is to know what you're eating and how much, and figuring out what is causing you to gain weight. If you're leaning more toward the second plan, do a trim — change some things on the plate.

Drop the big breakfast back to one egg, and get rid of the sausage and one slice of toast. That is still a big, yummy breakfast. For lunch, dump the chips and the Coke. At dinner, change the way you cook your veggies, drop the garlic bread, and have one glass of wine. As you can see, you don't have to count calories to know what's going to make you fat; look at the type and the amount of food you're eating and make changes to it.

How do you stay within your calorie-requirement range or shave off a few extra calories?

• Eat less at mealtimes; cut a quarter off your plate, and stick to the right serving sizes (see below).

• Don't eat as much in between meals – have no more than two snacks over the day, and make at least one a piece of fresh fruit.

• Stop drinking your calories.

• Don't nibble or graze on food all day.

• Move more: Add another 15 to 30 minutes a day onto your normal routine.

• Cut back on eating food you don't know all the ingredients of or how it's prepared (e.g., packaged food, fast food, restaurant/pub meals).

Don't worry about the calories — they will sort themselves out. Think more about the food you're eating, and really look at it.

It's not just food portions that have increased; plate, bowl, and cup sizes have as well. In the early 1990s, the standard size of a dinner plate increased from 25 to 30 cm (10 to 12 in.); cup and bowl sizes also increased.

What's the deal with food labels?

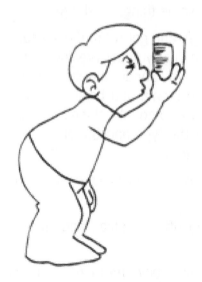

As I mentioned in Chapter 1: My Big Fat Rant, food isn't like cigarettes and doesn't come with graphic horror pictures on the pack. If it did, we'd put it down and run a mile. In fact, with food packaging, it's the opposite: Food comes with pretty, yummy, fresh pictures, regardless of what's inside the product. We have to sort it out for ourselves, but it's not as hard as the diet industry and media lead us to believe.

I like to read books and newspapers, but when it comes to reading my food, I'm bored to tears. Many of the food and diet experts tell us we should be spending extra time in the supermarkets reading the labels on the food products we're buying.

On the long list of all the things I want to do in my life, I'm afraid spending more time in the supermarket doesn't make it into the top 1,000.

I don't know if this is just a me thing, but the two most important things I should take into the supermarket are the things I always forget: My recycling bags and reading glasses.

I end up squinting at the back of packets and cans of foods to see how far up the list the chemicals are, and it's all a blur. I tend to try and go for the foods that don't have a label, as I figure they must be additive-free, so out I go with cauliflower and a bag of apples. Actually, maybe forgetting the specs is the key to losing weight — if you can't see or read the label, don't buy it!

Food manufacturers are required by law to list the true ingredients inside their products and the percentages of each, as well as provide nutritional information about that product. The exceptions are herbs and spices, mineral water, tea and coffee with nothing else added, food that is not packaged (i.e. fresh food), food that is made at point of sale (i.e. bread at the bakery), and food that comes in very small packaging, like gum and breath mints (though many companies opt to add lists to these products as well).

Packaged food and drinks are covered with labels, claims, and information, but there are really only two types of labels on food products that you need to be aware of:

1. Nutritional-information panel

2. Ingredients list

The nutritional-information panel is the breakdown of the calories and food groups. The list generally goes like this:

Energy (calories/kilojoules)
Total fat and saturated fat (the not-so-good fat)
Protein
Carbohydrates and sugars
Fibre
Salt

The values are usually per 100 g and often there will be another value that is the recommended serving size in grams.

The recommended serving size is at the discretion of the manufacturer, so it can be very different across products; even the same type of product or different brands can have different serving sizes on the labels. The biggest discrepancies can be found in oats and muesli, with some recommended serving sizes twice the size of others. Another culprit is chips and crisps, with one brand's serving being 19 g and others stating a recommended serving of 45 g., packaged popcorn can range from 15 to 100 g.

Serving sizes on yoghurt range from 100–200 g, and frozen packaged meals are all over the shop, ranging from 220–440 g a serving, depending on which brand you go with. As you can see, it's all very confusing to us consumers.

None of this means anything to me unless I can see that amount on my plate or in my bowl. On a muesli box once, I saw the serving size was 45 g, and when I got home, I realised that serving didn't even cover the bottom of my cereal bowl — it was about a quarter of a cup. I think it was a serving size for a mouse.

Lazy Tips for packet reading

No. 1 reading rule: Don't even bother reading the front of your food, as it's one big advertisement for the product. Labels at the front claiming "Low Fat", "Low Salt", "No Sugar", "High Fibre" may be correct, but how do you know for sure? Turn the package over and look at its official labels — they're not allowed to talk up or lie about the product.

Nutrition-information panel

Energy: This is the calories or kilojoules per 100 g or serving. For the energy label, go with the recommended serving size, not the 100 g. You need to know the amount you're going to eat and the serving size — and if you plan to eat two servings, double all the figures.

I suggest if you are going to study up on food, this is the best start, as it's no good knowing all the figures if you're eating three or more servings or more than 100 g.

I can usually visualise cup sizes, so this is what I think of when I see gram measurements: 120 g is usually half a cup; the 100 g on the label is less than that, so it's not much (240 g for a cup).

Liquid measurements are similar: 125 ml to half a cup and 250 ml to a cup; four cups to a litre.

Once again, go with the serving size. If the serving on the packet says 120 g and you know quite well you eat it by the cup, then double that figure.

For the rest of the list, use the 'per 100 g' and follow these guidelines. And if you get really confused, invest in a good set of kitchen scales and work it out yourself.

Protein: If there is any protein in the food, it's listed here per 100 g. You'll see this figure on products like meats, eggs, fish, legumes, and vegetarian options. Most of us get plenty of protein in our diets, but some people don't get enough.

People are 57% more likely to be obese if their friends are obese.

Fat: There are often two figures here: total fat and saturated fat.

Avoid foods where the saturated fat (see fats in Chapter 11) is more than half the total-fat figure or over 5 g per 100 g. Low saturated fat is under 1.5 g per 100 g.

If the total fat is more than 20 g per 100 g, this is high in fat; less than 3 g per 100 g is low (that's good).

Carbohydrates and sugar: Like fat, often carbohydrates and sugar are listed separately, and then a total figure is given. Carbohydrates include the starches found in foods like breads, pasta, and rices. Then there are natural sugars often found in fruit. And then there are the added sugars. It all adds up to total sugar, but it's always worth noticing the products that have more added sugar than natural sugar or starches.

If the total sugar is over 15 g per 100 g, that is a high sugar content. If you're watching your sugar intake or trying to lose weight, your sugar label should be under 5 g per 100 g.

And don't be fooled by the 0 fat on high-sugared foods, or the big banner on the front saying "No Fat" or "Low Fat" and think, *Well, this is good — at least it's only sugar and no fat.* They're referring to it having no oils or butters, but it's the sugars in this food that have all the calories, and it's too many of these things that make you fat, regardless of what label they're listed under. Go back to the top and look at the energy per serving.

Salt: This one gets slipped in on 90% of food, and in lots of cases, you'll be stunned at what foods have salt added. If the label says there is 1.5 g of salt per 100 g or 0.6 g of sodium, it sounds low, but that is a high salt content. Avoid these! Low salt is under 0.3 g, or 0.1 g of sodium per 100 g.

Fibre: This one is not always listed, as there may be no fibre content to report in many foods. So just seeing it on the list with a figure next to it is a good thing, and the higher the figure, the better. Fibre in our diets is always good.

Ingredients label

The ingredients in a product must be listed in descending order, so at the top will be the ingredient that weighs the most and the last thing on the list is the one that weighs the least. If an ingredient makes up less than 5% of the total product, it doesn't have to be listed.

If the front of your packet says "Strawberry Jam" and has a picture of yummy strawberries, but when you turn it over the ingredients label has water and sugar listed first with strawberry lower down, you're spreading strawberry-flavoured sugar on your toast.

The ingredients list includes water so often you'll usually see that nearer to the top of the list. Often an ingredient is on the list and given an overall percentage as well. This is the case with canned fruits or vegetables or other packaged fruit and vegetable products. If you're buying an apple pie and see "apples (25%)", it means a quarter of the pie contains real apples. When my mother made an apple pie, I'd say 75% of it was apples — that's a big difference. This is done to ensure that when a product boasts that it contains a fruit or vegetable and has the ingredient in its name, that most of it is made up of that food, and not just the fresh picture on the front of the packet.

You may often see a product that calls itself fruit in the name, but on the back, you find there is not fruit, but fruit flavour — which has no nutritional value at all and doesn't count as a fruit serving.

Another good time to check the ingredients label is when the food is advertised as having whole grains or being high in fibre. Whole grains should be among the top three ingredients. The nutrition-information panel should also have fibre listed, as the two go hand in hand.

The important things to note about the ingredients list are:

• The first three ingredients are what you're really eating, so make sure they match the product you think you're buying.

• The longer the list, the more processing, additives, and colourings there are, so look for shorter lists.

• Be aware of the sugar list. There could be five different styles of sugar on the label; anything ending in –ose is usually a sugar, and starches (corn), honey, and sweeteners are all forms of sugar. Add these up to get the total amount of sugar. All those little percentages could add up to match the main ingredient.

• Similar to sugar, all those different names of fats and oils add up. "Partially hydrogenated oil" is the big term for trans-fat — that's the one we should be reducing in our diets, so keep an eye out for it, because it crops up a lot!

• Lots of words you don't understand usually mean chemicals or preservatives. This tells you the degree of processing the food in the product has gone through to get into the packet. These things may be on the bottom of the list, but being there means lots of work has been done on that food. There are over 3,000 artificial additives that can be used in food, and I have no intention of listing them here! You'll know one if you can't pronounce it or it sounds like it was made in a test tube.

Lazy label-reading

Here are my quick tips if you haven't time to read or have forgotten your glasses:

• Five ingredients on a list is plenty; any more than that and it's over-processed or made up of things you don't need to be eating.

• If you're looking to cut back on sugar, don't buy products that feature it in the top three ingredients or contain over 15 g per 100 g (for drinks, 7.5 g per 100 ml). If the product has a natural fruit percentage, then you can go to 25 g per 100 g.

• If you're looking to reduce your fat intake, look for products that have less than 20 g per 100 g and check that the saturated fat is under 5 g per 100 g.

• If you're trying to increase whole grains, don't take the claims on the front of the product as gospel: Make sure it shows on the label. Over 5 g per 100 g is high in fibre.

Serving sizes

It's no good going on about the facts and figures of food and not knowing what those figures are based on. As you can tell from the lists above, it's about weight per grams, and the serving sizes are randomly plucked out of the air by manufacturers.

Serving sizes are growing just like we are. But the figures stay the same, so if you're eating a piece of steak that equals three servings, you have to multiply everything in that steak by three (P.S. Three pieces of steak for dinner nightly will make you fat).

A serving of orange juice is 125 ml. If you pour that into your usual tall glass, it will only fill it halfway. Therefore, if you have one of your glasses of orange juice, you're really having two servings, which could be an extra 100 calories a day. And you know the drill by now: That's 700 extra calories a week, which adds 4.5 kg a year — and that's just from mucking up one serving size of a drink!

Let's have a general look at what we're required to eat in a day:

Food groups

Cereals

Men: Six to 10 servings; Women: Four to eight servings.

• The cereal group includes breads, cereals, rices, and noodles.
• A serving is:
  o two slices of bread
  o one roll
  o a cup of cooked rice or pasta
  o half a cup of muesli

Vegetables

Men and women: Five servings.

• The vegetable group includes leafy vegetables, starchy vegetables, and legumes.

- A serving is:
  - o   one medium white potato
  - o   half a medium sweet potato
  - o   one medium parsnip
  - o   one cup of green leafy vegetables/lettuce
  - o   half a cup of all other vegetables (e.g., beans, lentils, peas, corn)

Fruit

Men and women: Two servings.

A serving is:

- One medium piece of fruit (e.g., apple, pear, orange, banana)
- Two pieces of a smaller fruit (e.g., apricots, plums, figs)
- Eight small strawberries or 20 grapes
- One cup of (sugar-free) canned fruit
- 125 ml of freshly squeezed, no-sugar-added juice

Dairy

Men and women: Two servings.

- The dairy group includes milk, yoghurt, cheese, and dairy alternatives.
- A serving is:
  - o   250 ml of milk
  - o   40 g or two slices of cheese
  - o   200 g (a small tub) of yoghurt
  - o   250 ml of soymilk

A 2013 study in Britain showed 86 % of UK workers are shortening their life expectancy by an average of four years due to their sedentary lifestyles.

Meat, fish, poultry, and alternatives

Men and women: One serving.

A serving is:

• 70 to 100 g of cooked meat or chicken (half a cup of cooked mince, two small chops, or two slices of roast meat)

• 2 small eggs

• 80 to 120 g of cooked fish or seafood

Extras

We're also allowed one to three extras per day. I could be opening a big can of worms, but here are just a few extra serving sizes:

• One small slice of cake

• Two sweet biscuits

• Half a chocolate bar

• 60 g or 1 Tbsp. honey or jam

• 30 g (small packet) of chips or crisps

• One can of soft drink

• 200 ml glass of wine

• 400 ml of regular or 600 ml of light beer

• 30 ml of spirits with mixer

• one scoop of ice cream

• 1 Tbsp. of butter

• Small slice of pizza

• Half a meat pie

• 2 Tbsp. cream or mayonnaise

• 10 hot chips

Now that you know the serving sizes and food groups, it all makes sense now, doesn't it?

Yeah, right!

Have you seen the varieties of bread lately? One slice could be 10 cm x 10 cm and 1 cm thick, but then there are the huge slabs measuring 15 cm x 15 cm with nearly double the thickness. Sorry — the one serving mentioned above is for the little skinny ones. The bread roll mentioned is 50 g, and not much bigger than a soup roll. Most rolls that we have for lunch or buy filled would be regarded as large (a serving and a half).

The serving of meat suggested would be very hard to find at the butcher or supermarket, as the piece you see would have to be trimmed to half or a third (maybe even a quarter). The serving of meat should be the size of the palm of your hand (without your fingers, I'm afraid). And then there's the thickness: Go for less than 2 cm. If you like a thick, juicy piece of meat, then go for a smaller area size. It used to be common to assume a chicken breast was a serving, but that's not the case — chickens, like humans, are getting bigger boobs! So half a chicken breast is more likely a serve these days.

We need a system for when we shop. Below is how I judge the size of things for myself:

• If a piece of meat is the size of my whole hand, it's two servings. If it's a thick, chunky piece, it's three. In my mind's eye, I've already cut it up and know it will feed two or three people that evening.

• I haven't seen a small chicken breast in a long, long time, so I assume a whole breast is two servings; that is good enough for me. If I'm using it in a stir-fry or casserole for two or three people, one large breast is enough.

• I allow more for fish, but still, some of those fillets look like they came straight off the side of a white pointer! I would quarter up an extra-long fillet. Salmon is easy, as it's often sliced to the right serving size and I could use my hand rule for it. For prawns (shrimp), a serving is six large or 10 to 12 small ones.

Cookbooks in the 1970s had recipes recommended to serve six people. The same recipes in the present era are now recommended to feed four.

• Cheese is a tough one, as you buy it by the block and then just keep on eating away at it until it's time to go buy a new one. For one serving size, think of a box of matches (or, if you've forgotten what that looks like, a pack of Tic Tacs). If it's sliced cheese you're eating, that's easy: Two slices per serving.

• Dips are another tricky one. I've been known to eat a whole tub on my own, and that's not counting the cheese sticks I used to scoop it out with. However, most tubs contain two to four servings. So now when I open a tub on my own, I know that half has to be left when I finish. If you share it among two or three people, you're fine; however, you still have the crackers to count as well.

• While we're at it, how many biscuits are suitable to go with your dip? Dry biscuits and rice crackers fall under your bread allowances. Five medium crackers (each about the size of the circle your thumb and index finger make together) are about the same as a slice of bread, and as two slices of bread are a serving, you can have 10 of those crackers with your dip or cheese. For rice crackers, you can double that and have 20. As you know, these biscuits come in many shapes and sizes, and also come in a range of flavours with oils and salts added, so you'll need to have a quick check of your labels with dried biscuits.

• Fluids are easy if you know your cup measurement, which is 250 ml. However, you are probably best to know your 1.5 cup measurement or even 2 cup, as that is what most drinks are canned or bottled at. A can or small bottle is 375 ml. Cartons of flavoured milk come in 500 ml, which is two serves of dairy. But goodness knows how much sugar is in them; you'll have to sort that out by the calorie or sugar count.

• For yoghurt, the serving size is a small tub — that bit's easy. When I buy yoghurt, I buy a small tub of plain Greek yoghurt, halve it, and add my own fresh fruit. I heard you gasp at the mention of "Greek yoghurt" — yes, it's rich and not low in calories or fat, but my strategy is to have half a serving with a serving of fruit. It fills me up, tastes great, and I have half left for tomorrow.

• An ice-cream serving is the good-old-fashioned scoop; luckily, that hasn't grown over the years. If you don't have a scoop, it's half a cup. It's not much, so add a serving of fresh fruit!

• Things like soups, stews, and casseroles are easy — you just bung in the right serving sizes of everything and double, triple, or quadruple based on the amount of people joining in the meal (i.e. three servings of veggies and one serving of meat per person). The only problem with this is the sauces and creams we add, which should be based on the nutritional information label. Again, try to stick to the right servings.

• With butter, margarine, oil, mayonnaise, cream, and all those other rich goodies . . . now, you know this is not going to be much. With butter, visualise those little wrapped portions hotels give you; for oil and mayonnaise, think of a tablespoon. For double cream and whipped cream, a serving is 2 Tbsp.; for light cream, 4 Tbsp.

• Rice and pasta serving sizes are when cooked. Dried rice and pasta double when cooked, so if you've been serving yourself a cup of dried rice a night (which is two cups of cooked), maybe that's what you've been doing wrong all these years! For two people, put one cup of dried rice in the pot; it will turn into two servings when cooked. If you want to know what the serving looks like on your plate, it should be the size of a tennis ball. Dried pasta is similar: Half a dried cup is a serving, and when it's cooked, it should be one cup. If you're putting on a pasta sauce, depending on the ingredient, one cup is a good serving.

After 50 years of eating, reading, and working mostly in the health industry, I can broadly assess what is going to make me fat, sluggish, or energised, and what is good for me. And I don't need a calculator, app, or degree in food science to tell me. When I'm looking to buy food, looking at it is usually the first thing I do.

Overweightness and obesity are the fifth leading risk for global deaths. At least 2.8 million adults die each year as a result of being overweight or obese. In addition, 44% of the diabetes burden, 23% of the ischaemic-heart-disease burden, and between 7 and 41% of certain cancer burdens are attributable to overweight and obesity.

Viewing rules for food and drink

Not-so-good choices have the following characteristics:

• It's in a packet, with a long list of ingredients.

• It's a meat/poultry/fish covered in bread-like crumbs or a yellow/golden batter.

• It's called a vegetable but you can't see what type, as it's covered in a white sauce or melted cheese.

• It's drowned in a creamy white sauce.

• It looks like it has come out of a meaningful relationship with a deep fryer.

• There are visible signs of white fat or fatty skin.

• It's crispy brown and leaves a greasy residue on your fingers.

• It's served to you by a teenager with headset on, in a paper bag, out of a window while you're seated in your car.

• It's very colourful and not a fruit or vegetable.

• It's wrapped in pastry.

• It's coated in sugar.

• It's a brightly coloured or bubbly drink.

• It's covered in melted cheese.

Here are my viewing rules for things I eat on a daily basis, and are healthier choices:

• It's a fruit or vegie that came out of the ground or off a tree in the last month.

• It's not in a packet with writing all over it.

• If it's meat, it's red; chicken, it's pink; fish, it's white, pink, or clear. Regardless of type, it's not coated in anything (breadcrumbs, batter, oils, etc.).

• If it's bread, it's wholegrain.

• If it's in a glass, it's water (with the exception of the occasional wine!).

Here's what my taste buds tell me about food, and what I tell myself about it:

- "It is SO sweet!" Nothing that is natural can taste that sweet, so it has sugar added. This applies to packaged food and drinks.

- "The first thing I taste is salt." This means salt is added to the finished product, and probably inside it as well.

- "It's smooth and creamy." This is great, but don't have too much, as it's surely made with butter or full-fat cream.

- "Lots of different flavours jump out at me." This is fine if I added those wonderful flavours myself or I know the restaurant chef lovingly did, but if it isn't from either of us, then they're probably artificial, added flavours.

Use good-old-fashioned common sense

In our technical, electronic, and complicated world, many of us have lost faith in our gut instincts and common sense when it comes to food selection. We have to turn on an app, refer to the latest diet book, or look up a calorie counter every time we encounter a new food product or meal.

We second guess ourselves so much that we take the easy option of buying pre-packaged, tasteless meals: The ones that now fill our supermarket freezers or can be delivered to our doors. They have the exact serving size, calories, and fat that we need to lose weight. The food manufactures love it and lead us by the nose, telling us that all the preparation and planning of meals has been sorted — all we need to do is buy lots of packets, take them home, stick one in the oven each evening, and dinner is ready.

A study published in the American Journal of Preventive Medicine found that when people were given larger bowls and spoons, they served themselves larger portions of ice cream and tended to eat the whole portion.

I have a few problems with this way of eating:

1. We get used to eating like this, so when it comes to preparing our own meals or eating out, we have no idea of serving sizes or how to get a good balance of nutrients on our plates.

2. Packaged meals are never as nutritious and wholesome as fresh vegetables, fruit, and meats we can prepare for ourselves.

3. Our confidence with knowing the right way to prepare food and eat healthily decreases, and then we can't pass that good knowledge onto our kids.

4. Packaged meals can be bland and boring, and after a while our tastebuds adapt, so the pleasure of eating diminishes. It's often then we crave the strong flavours of sugar or salt to compensate.

5. If they're not filling us up or satisfying our nutritional needs, we add on things like bread, sweets, or cheese and crackers after our packaged meals — and those calories are not included on the side of that pack.

You don't need to be a chef to cook — we can all do it, and it's not our home cooking that is making us fat: It's the lack thereof. Eating out, getting food delivered, picking food up on the way home from work, or grabbing packets out of the freezer is all processed food. You don't know how it was prepared, and you probably know it's not the best nutritional choice.

We live this way because we think it's easier, faster, and cheaper. I am a self-confessed lazy person, but I still think cooking and preparing your own meals is faster, cheaper, less of a hassle, and healthier.

I can make soup or fish and salad in 10 minutes, steak and vegetables in 15, rice and pasta dishes in 20 to 30, and yes, I can even slap a roast in the oven. That may take two hours, but I've sat on my bum reading or watching telly while it cooks. See? Even a lazy sod like me can do it.

By the time you drive through the drive-thru, wait for the pizza guy, or defrost and cook all your packaged meal, I bet the times match mine above. So don't pull the time-strapped card on me — it can be done.

Lazy Bottom Line

• Unless you plan on counting calories the rest of your life, don't bother starting. Cut back meal sizes, sweet things, and greasy foods and you'll end up eating fewer calories. Move a bit more, and you'll burn off calories.

• Nutrition-information panels can be helpful when you're confused about what's in a packaged product. So have a quick squiz, but you don't have to read the label on every product you buy. And if you hate reading and feel guilty if you don't, buy the stuff with no writing on it — it's usually the best for you anyway.

• It's important to know serving sizes. Food is getting bigger and bulkier, and the number of calories in it grows as well. Most of us eat more than the serving size on the packet.

• Take back control of your food and eating. Buy fresh and cook for yourself and your family. The hype around pre-packaged meals being faster, easier and healthier is just that — all hype. You can prepare and cook meals quickly, have a go at it.

• Spend more time looking at the food you buy and go with your gut (no, not the one that is rumbling — your gut instinct).

In 1955, a beef patty in a fast-food hamburger weighed around 45 g (1.6 oz); now, the largest hamburger patty weighs 226 g (8 oz), an increase of 500%.

Chapter 11 – No Food is Bad

All food is good. There, I've said it.

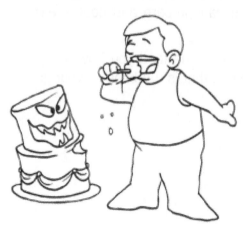

No food is evil, mean, or going to kill or poison you (unless it contains actual poison, of course!) Food is wonderful: It keeps us alive and brings lots of joy to our lives.

I know what you're thinking: Where's the "but"?

There's no "but". Sugar is brilliant — love it. Fats and oils? Bring 'em on! Carbs? Thrive on them. Protein: What a fantastic invention! The whole lot is what we need to survive, grow, and have lots of energy.

Yeah, I know you're still waiting for your "but", but I'm not giving it to you.

We need all of the above foods, and if you want figures, the daily breakdown is:

- 50 to 55% carbohydrates
- 20 to 25% fat
- 20 to 25% protein

All foods you consume should be the freshest, healthiest, most minimally processed choices. As you can see, carbs still rule and fats are allowed, regardless of all the hype and fads we're brainwashed with regularly.

I know we're getting fatter and maybe unhealthier; however, I don't like the way the experts are blaming food for the obesity crisis. Pitting each food group against one another, with each sugar variety in a different corner of the boxing ring along with the drama associated with food labelling, it doesn't help our attitude toward food and eating — it just adds to the confusion.

Food and food products have changed from our parents' and grandparents' days, but the food they ate hasn't disappeared. It's still there, growing in fields and on trees and bushes, and walking around in paddocks. Sure, it's served and packaged in a million more ways — some naturally, and some with so much stuff added you don't even know if it ever come out of the ground. However, food choices exist, and food is still there to be eaten in any state.

If there is a "but", it's "But there are so many choices, and I'm confused by them." Most of that confusion is generated by multinational food corporations, with their ambiguous food claims and labels, as well as the amount of information — good, bad, right, wrong — out there in the media, in books, and on the internet.

Bad foods? No such thing

I know I've gone on in other chapters about high-sugared foods (especially soft drinks) and low-fat foods that have chemicals in them to trick you into feeling satisfied and full, as well as the all the packaged foods out there. In Chapter 8: Rules, many of the rules are based on reducing or even stopping the consumption of some foods. But that still doesn't mean that food is bad or evil —

it simply means you may need to ease off it or stop eating it if it's causing you to put on weight or affecting your health.

If you are overweight or obese; have high blood pressure, diabetes, a heart condition, or a family history of any of these health problems; allergic to certain foods; in remission from cancer; or have had other illnesses and conditions that may reoccur over your lifetime, then yes, some foods will not be ideal — or good — for you.

However, many foods just get a bad rap. They also go in and out of fashion, depending on new scientific findings or a story the media has picked up and run with. Some foods are really good for you; others, not so good. But they're all there, under our noses, to be purchased and eaten. What are you going to do with all of these choices? Make your own: The right ones for you.

Below are a few things that have been in and out, and up and down on food charts and pyramids. Some get a bad rap; others are raved about as the new wonder foods. I've only included foods that many of my clients have asked me about (or have told me things about that I know are just crazy), so I'm going to get on my soapbox here and dispel a few food myths:

Alcohol

If you're a teetotaller, move on! But for the rest of you, stay tuned.

You can drink alcohol, but it is high in sugar and calories. If you drink too much, you'll put on weight.

Scientists (and red-wine lovers) claim some alcohol is good for your heart health and that you should drink it, but that still doesn't give you license to do so by the jug. The calorie content for most alcoholic drinks is as follows:

• Glass of wine (white or red), 250 ml: 178 calories

• Flute of champagne, 150 ml: 111 calories

> Overheard in a doctor's office: "It's not that diabetes, heart disease, and obesity run in your family — it's that no one runs in your family."

- Spirit with no mixer or low-calorie mixer: 117 calories (with mixer: 200 calories)
- Beer, per 100 ml: 35 to 45 calories
  - Pot or stubby of regular beer, 375 ml: 140 calories
  - Mid-strength beer, 375 ml: 103 calories
  - Light beer, 375 ml: 85 calories
- Bottle of cider, 375 ml: 161 calories
- Alcoholic pop-flavoured drink, 250 ml: 170 calories

Often, the extra calories and sugars come from ingredients put in drinks like cocktails, high-energy mixers, milk, and juices. The main problem with drinking calories is that they are empty; they don't fill you up, and you forget to include them as part of your eating plan.

You may eat healthy all day and watch or even count your calories, but if you don't include the couple of drinks you have a day or the big night out you have every weekend, you'll gain weight. Four alcoholic drinks a week that aren't calculated into the left side of your Lazy Loser scales and not worked off in the right side of the scales could make you gain 5 kg a year!

However, it's not just calories and weight gain that alcohol causes — it's now widely recognised by anti-cancer council authorities worldwide that the consumption of alcohol can lead to some cancers.

A very scary statistic is that 22% of breast cancers in Australia have been linked to alcohol consumption. The reason is that alcohol increases sex hormones, and high levels of oestrogen are a risk factor for breast cancer. Other cancer types alcohol is linked to are mouth, throat, oesophagus, and bowel.

It's not just one type of alcohol — any variety can be a risk. Cutting back alcohol consumption is advised, and experts recommended no more than two standard drinks a day. A standard drink contains 10gm of alcohol regardless of the type or size of the drink. Bear in mind one standard drink is only 100 ml (small glass) of wine or a 285 ml glass of full strength beer, so it's very easy to go over the recommended limit.

Bread

Bread is okay; however, we average six slices a day, which is a bit too much (I think two to four is plenty). Bread now comes in all shapes, sizes, and prices. The standard two slices are what we know from our school lunches: Two flat, white, thin, square slices of bread that if you held it up to the light you could see through! A standard roll is equivalent to two slices of bread.

Breads are now thicker and so large they sometimes don't even fit in the toaster. Often, in those cases, one slice is equal to two slices. And yes, if they're bigger and fatter, then it stands to reason they'll have more calories that make you bigger and fatter!

Take that into consideration when you plan your food intake. White bread is not evil, but it's not the best choice for fibre content; wholemeal, wholegrain, rye, and sourdough are all good choices. The new fancy breads — Turkish bread and focaccia-style breads — are usually white and have a lot more fat content and double or more the calories of normal bread. So once again, it's not bad — but if you're looking for healthy options or to lose weight, they're not the choice for you.

Although bread isn't bad for us, cutting back will save calories. Bread is fine as toast for breakfast and for sandwiches at lunch, but serving it at night alongside a full plate of dinner is an added extra you don't need.

Eggs

In my last book, "Lazy Runner", I got on my soapbox to stand up for the poor googy egg, and I'm going to repeat myself here.

The poor egg has had an absolute battering over the past 10 years, but please believe me when I say eggs are good for you. They're a fantastic food source. You can safely eat three eggs a day, yet the crazy egg scare has seen people reduce their intake to fewer than three eggs per week.

Eggs do not give you high cholesterol. If you do suffer from high cholesterol, you will be told to cut back on certain foods and eggs may be one of them, but if you have no cholesterol issues, eating eggs will not give you a high reading. Body builders eat up to 20 eggs a day, and it has been proven that it doesn't increase their bad-cholesterol count. Eggs are great for the right side of your Lazy Loser scales as well, as they're high in protein, and you need that to repair your muscles after intense exercise.

Another reason eggs are great is they fill you up; have a couple of scrambled or poached eggs in the morning, and I bet you're full until lunchtime. Like lots of food you prepare yourself, if depends on how you cook them and what you put on or in them, but a small egg has only 37 calories and an extra-large one has 85. And for goodness sake, leave the yolk in — it's the best bit!

Drinks

Flavoured drinks are one of the biggest problems with excess sugar intake, excess calories and, in turn, society's obesity problems. A drink is never really considered a meal or even a snack, and we tend not to count it in our daily intake of calories or even as food intake.

There are so many drinks out there now, but basically they're all the same: High in sugar and empty calories. And I know you're going to tell me you have the low- or zero-calorie drinks, but they still feed your craving for sugar and, in turn, keep you wanting more sweet stuff.

As a marathon runner and coach, I recommend sports drinks when training because I think they contain all the right elements to replace what you lose when running and working out. However, they should only be consumed before or after a run, or when carb loading for a big event like a half or full marathon. I see kids drinking them on their way to school or people having them with their lunches, like a normal drink. This means they are consuming lots of sugar and carbs they're probably not going to use or burn off over the course of the day.

And it's not just sports drinks: It's also all these wonderful new trendy juices out there that claim to be worth two to three servings of fruit or veggies. They don't tell you they probably also have 10 to 20 servings of sugar. If you want two to three servings of fruit, eat some fruit — don't drink it. It will be healthier for you, fill you up, and probably contain fewer calories. I say drink water and eat food.

Chocolate

Is chocolate the new be-all, end-all wonder food that's so good for you that you can eat it by the bucket? Or is this just the wishful thinking of all the chocolate lovers around the world?

The truth is that cocoa (the basis of all milk or dark chocolate, not white chocolate) has flavonoids, which are anti-oxidants that are good for us. One study that compared the total antioxidant activity in single servings of cocoa, green tea, black tea, and red wine scored cocoa markedly higher than the rest.

But be aware that fruits and veggies have flavonoids that are good for you and have fewer calories. Yeah, I hear you: "They don't taste as good, though!"

The flavonoids in chocolate are called flavanols and procyanidins, and they have a powerful antioxidant affect. This rise in antioxidant levels helps protect us from damage to the heart and blood vessels, and also guards our DNA from damage that can lead to cancer.

The more cocoa in your chocolate, the more antioxidants there are. This is why dark chocolate is classified as better (but cocoa is still in milk chocolate). You may think an easy way to get the benefits are to drink hot cocoa every night, but that doesn't work: The cocoa we use for drinking chocolate is usually the Dutch type, and its processing strips the good flavonoids out.

Chocolate, like eggs, does not cause high cholesterol, as the good fats in it don't affect those levels. However, the sugar and excess eating of it can, and like with eggs, if your cholesterol was high, you'd need to look at your chocolate intake. A small piece of dark chocolate is about 50 calories, but most chocolate bars are over 200 calories, and usually have more stuff added to the chocolate.

And is chocolate addictive, like us chocoholics claim it to be? Most scientists say no — that it does contain things that make us feel good, warm, and fuzzy, but it doesn't have addictive agents. So we do have control over how often we eat it, and how much we eat!

A study comparing eating habits today with those of 20 years ago found that participants poured themselves about 20% more cereal and 30 % more milk now.

We like the taste, crave it, and feel better when we eat it, but all those things are not considered symptoms of an addiction.

Meat

Unless you're a vegetarian and have issues with eating baby animals or it's against your religion to eat certain types of meat, eat meat. All meat is good for you: Lamb, beef, pork, kangaroo, mincemeats, offal — the whole lot — but you need to buy it fresh and trim visible fat. If you're buying mince, you can usually see the white fatty content. I find when buying mince, you should choose the high quality grade. It may be more expensive, but overall it's still a cheap meal. Once again, it's not the actual piece of meat that's bad — it's the serving sizes, or what we put on top of it. Most people have too large a serving. The steaks you see in restaurants that cover half the plate? That's probably two to three servings.

A serving of steak or any other meat should be the size of the palm of your hand, and about a third of what's on your plate. Creamy sauces are the fattening things, so go for tomato-based sauces and toppings. If you're having a roast, the serving should be two slices of meat.

The main problem with meat is buying it out and not preparing it yourself — you have no idea what sort of meat is going into the hamburgers you buy, or how your meat is prepared or cooked when you order out. But at home you have lots of control, so buy it and cook it.

Red meat is a good source of iron and also contains protein, levels of creatine, minerals such as zinc and phosphorus, and vitamins such as niacin, vitamin B12, thiamin, and riboflavin. Red meat is also the richest source of alpha lipoic acid, a powerful antioxidant.

However, the western world is mad for meat and tends to eat far too much of it, too regularly. High consumption of red meat is still connected to heart disease, even if it's a lean variety of red meat. If you eat red meat daily, try replacing a few servings a week with a white meat, fish, or vegetarian dish.

Processed meats (bacon, ham, and salami) are not a healthy choice, and have also been linked to bowel cancer. Plus, they're usually processed and a lot higher in fat and calories, so if you are consuming them often, they'll make you fat!

Potatoes

Potatoes are vegetables, so they can't be bad, right? The poor spud has become a veggie victim — not because it's unhealthy or fattening, but more often because of the way it's prepared or what's put on top of it. A boiled potato is good. A potato cut up into little pieces and deep fried? Not as good.

If you're adding oil or butter or baking your potatoes in creamy sauces and adding grated cheese on top, you can't blame the spud for making you fat. One or two potatoes steamed, boiled, or baked in their jackets are low fat; they're very filling, and a great source of carbohydrates, which equate to energy.

And if you like your potatoes made into a creamy mash, you don't need lots of butter and cream. Try mashing them with skim milk and chives or extra virgin olive oil: Same result with far fewer calories.

Vegetables

While I'm on the humble spud, I may as well mention all his buddies. Vegetables are all good, and yes, the recommended dose is 5 servings a day. It sounds like a lot, but again, it's the serving size that catches us out. A serving size of peas is 3 Tbsp. — that is not much. A whole ear (cob) of corn is three servings, not one. Therefore, at dinner, if you have 3 Tbsp. of peas, a corn cob, and half a cup of cooked carrots, there are your five servings for the day.

Like the spud, often it's not the five veggie servings that are making you fat — it's how you're preparing them. You could easily get your five veggie servings into a stir-fry dish by using some olive oil to fry them and making a light sauce using soy sauce, balsamic vinegar,

When you upsize your meal deal at a fast-food chain from a burger, drink, and fries to a burger, a large drink, and large fries, you've only increased the cost by 16 per cent, but the calorie count increased by 40%.

Lazy Loser

and honey. Or you could add a rich pasta sauce made with cream, butter, and cheese. Don't blame the veggies if you're eating the latter all the time.

All vegetables are good for you, and the majority are low in fat and sugar and high in fibre, vitamins, and minerals. But guess what? Vegetables still have calories. Most are low in calories and some have more calories than others, but the calories still mean they're going into the left side of your Lazy Loser scales. You may love vegetables and eat them by the bucket, but anything that has calories can be overeaten and make you fat. It's the law of the food jungle, and you should never forget it when it comes to eating — no matter how healthy that food is.

Last word on vegetables: Many people tell me they hate vegetables and can't eat them. To which I reply, "Are you serious? Out of the hundreds of vegetable varieties, you can't find one you can tolerate?" Lazy Loser is not a diet. It's about staying fit, well, and healthy all your life. Not eating any vegetables will not put you in this category, so you may as well ditch this book now if you can't eat any vegetables.

I know it sounds like a contradiction — as I'm always saying you shouldn't eat anything you don't like — but you need to return to your vegetable drawing board and go through them all until you find some vegetables you do like. Make soups — no, not creamy fattening ones. A soup made with pumpkin, carrots, onions, skim milk, and a few herbs and spices is delicious — and that's three veggies down. Make stews and casseroles or stir-fries; the meat juices in them seep into the veggies, making them taste great. You don't need to be chewing on raw carrots and celery all day to get your daily dose of veggies in.

I never served my kids plain white rice when we were having rice with a meal — I always threw in a couple of cups of cooked veggies like peas, corn, diced capsicum, grated carrots, or diced onion. They got so used to seeing all the bright colours in their rice that if we went out for dinner and plain rice was served, they'd look at it and think, *Boring!* If you're a non-veggie-eater, it's a bad habit you've gotten into, so start changing it. Introduce veggies gradually in clever ways until you're in the habit of eating them.

Loser Tale

This is a good one for veggie haters, and especially parents of children who are heading in that direction. When my two boys were little, they were mostly good with eating their veggies, but one hated peas and one liked peas while one hated corn and the other loved corn. Each night, I had to cook piles of veggies (which their father and I ate), and then one little plate would have carrots, corn, and broccoli and one little plate would have carrots, peas, and broccoli.

I got tired of the extra vegetable preparation, so one evening, on the carrots, corn, and broccoli plate, I put one little pea, and on the carrots, peas, and broccoli plate, I placed one little kernel of corn.

Well, you can imagine the cries from each respondent. I just said, "Oh dear, it looks like one little pea and corn jumped plates! Oh, well, you have to eat it — no sweets if you don't eat all your veggies." Mind you, this was back in the day before blackmail and bribery were outlawed from the child-rearing program.

Of course they each ate the one lonely little pea and corn kernel. Well, what do you know — the next night, two little peas had jumped onto the corn plate and two little corn kernels had jumped ship to the pea plate. "Oh well, just eat them up for ice cream." Every night, there was a little mutiny of peas and corn, until I had nearly forgotten who preferred what (well, maybe not quite — I always put a bit less of the hated veggie on each plate, as I didn't want to push my luck).

They are both men now and I know one still isn't keen on peas and one not so fond of corn, but the point is they eat both. Moral of this tale: If you don't like veggies, treat yourself like a kid. Start with one tiny piece of a hated veggie: Hide it on the plate or slip it into your favourite recipe. Before you know it, you'll wonder what the fuss was about.

Fruit

This is my favourite. No rules needed for me with fruit: I love it. Once again though, there are calories in there. The rule you can never have too much of a good thing does not apply to fruit. The two serves a day is easy. No preparation or cooking, great for snacks, easy to take and eat anywhere.

Fruit is mostly low in calories, though, not as low as veggies, and some can be higher up than you think: Avocados, mangos, bananas, dates, and figs are some higher-calorie fruit varieties. That doesn't mean you can't have them — it just means that number of calories is going into the left hand side of your Lazy Loser scales, and if you haven't got enough energy output in the right side, you can gain weight from eating too much fruit.

Fruit is great in all forms, but fresh is best. The next best is snap frozen, which is a great option for when fruits (such as berries) are out of season. Be aware that tinned fruit has been processed before it gets into the can, and could have added sugar in the syrup. You can test this theory out for yourself: Stew some fruit (like apples, pears, or peaches), don't add anything, and then have a taste. It can be pretty tart and sour — even the juice. Then have it cooked or stewed from a can — quite sweet. Hmmm . . . I wonder why?

Be very aware of choosing dried fruit. It tastes great and is a good snack, but has lots more calories than fresh fruit and is never as filling.

Fats and oils

Like eggs, fats were shunned and abused during the '90s, but most people now accept that all fats are not bad — in fact, some do more good than harm.

Good fats are those containing omega-3 sources, which can be found in fish. Other (notice I didn't say bad) fats are the trans fats in fast-food meals and packaged foods.

Fats play a very important role in keeping the body healthy. If you're not overweight, you should not try to decrease your good-fat intake, as you could cause an imbalance to normal body functions that rely on a healthy fat intake.

We need fats for hormone function, body support and protection, insulation, and temperature regulation. Not to mention our brain is 60% fat, and it needs that amount to think and remember.

The problem with fats is sorting out the best fats to eat. When you read the nutritional labels on food, you'll often see three types of fats listed:

- Trans fat
- Saturated fat
- Unsaturated fat

The first one is the one to avoid or cut back on if you're overweight or have any health risks, like high cholesterol. The second one is okay in smaller quantities, and the third is the healthiest and best choice.

Unfortunately, it's often the first two that are at the top of the list on fast, processed, and prepared foods. The best fat, unsaturated, is made up of two types: Monounsaturated and polyunsaturated. Both are good for your heart health. Good fats are sourced from olive and canola oil, nuts, seeds, oily fish, and avocados. Not-so-good fats are found in vegetable oils, margarines, and most fast and processed foods.

Trans fats are not the best choice for anyone. It doesn't matter if you're skinny, fat, or of a normal weight: Continuing to eat too many of these fats will have a negative impact on your health.

The best thing about fats is that they fill you up, often leaving you satisfied for much longer and, as a result, you eat less. Fat is a denser food, due to its high-calorie rate (9 calories per gram), as opposed to carbohydrates and protein, which have 4 calories per gram. You should aim to make fat 20 to 25% of your daily diet.

Nuts

I've stuck these little gems in this chapter, as I love them and think they're so good for us. Most nuts are high in fat. I can hear you hollering at me: "How you can say they're good for us!?" But the fats in nuts are as I mentioned above: Good fats. Once again, the problem is in serving sizes, but eating nuts daily is good for you and can be done without getting fat.

Nuts have the best type of fats — unsaturated and monounsaturated — which makes them good for heart health. But they also contain vitamin E and are rich in protein, fibre, magnesium, copper, phosphorus, potassium, selenium, and folate. Plus, they taste good and fill you up.

Serving sizes are important and each nut can differ, but I say 10 to 20 nuts for a snack is about right. Count them out and put them in a bowl so you don't over eat them.

I eat lots of nuts. "How can you do that and stay the right weight?", you ask? Easy: It fits in with my scales — they are in the left side, and the right side is balanced. If I was putting on weight, I'd probably look at my nut consumption and maybe adjust it, but at this stage, it's not an issue, so I'm sticking with my nut habit.

Salt

This one has really taken a hammering over the past few years. And you probably say, "My parents and grandparents added salt to everything, and they were fine." Yes, but that's because they prepared everything they ate; even the salt they added into their cooking and at the table would never match the salt that's slipped into 90% of the processed food we eat now.

Salt, known as sodium in the body, is an essential part of bodily functions. The average body has approximately 75,000 mg of sodium; that adds up to 11 Tbsp. of salt, and it makes up 0.4% of the human body. Our kidneys regulate the amount of salt in our systems. If we go overboard on salt in our diets, it's often removed through our urine. However, some people retain salt in their blood, and this is the common cause of high blood pressure.

You should consume no more than 2,000 mg of salt a day, with 1,600 being the recommended amount for an adult. This is equivalent to 4 g of salt a day, but most of us consume 10 g or more!

The colours red, yellow, and orange stimulate hunger. Think about the colours of all the fast-food outlets and their logos — see the connection?

There are easy ways to cut back on your salt intake:

• Prepare your own meals — do not buy processed or packaged foods.

• Don't add salt at the table, and add only sparingly when cooking.

• Opt for low-salt/sodium products.

Remember: The more food you prepare for yourself, the easier it is to control what goes into it — and salt is right at the top of that control list.

Salt is an acquired taste, and after years of eating it, our palates tell us things without salt are tasteless. If you reduce your salt intake, you reduce your habit for salt, and after a while all the wonderful new tastes will come through. I never buy salted nuts, as I love the natural taste of nuts; if I have salted nuts when I'm out, all I taste is salt.

You're probably thinking salt has no calories and isn't fattening, but that's not the issue. Salt makes you thirsty, so you drink more alcohol or sweet drinks. Salt on snacks is also morish, so you can't stop at one. More food and drink = more calories.

Sugar

I could just say "Read the one above" or "Ditto", as sugar is nearly the same problem as salt. Once again, our parents added lots of sugar to things they dished up to us — cereals, stewed fruit, cups of tea, etc. — and that wasn't so good, but boy it was probably a lot less sugar than anything we get in packets and containers now.

I don't know how many spoons of sugar my mum put on my Weetabix, but I don't think it was five (as that's what many of the packaged cereals have added per bowl). Even some of the ones we think are good for us have 2 or 3 tsp. of sugar per serving.

Sugar is known as sucrose, and consists of 50% fructose and 50% glucose. Sweet foods such as desserts, cakes, chocolate, and sweetened beverages such as carbonated soft drinks, sports drinks, and so on, contain large quantities of added fructose. Fruit juice is also high in fructose. So, as you can see, it's the packaged foods we're buying that are the problem, as we can't see the sugar content. But rest assured it's there — and in quantities that would stagger you if you were putting the same amount in your own food from the sugar bowl.

Tips to reduce your sugar intake are:

• Don't start the day with a high-sugared breakfast; if you like cereal, make your own from healthy grains, or have porridge. The earlier in the day you start eating sugar, the earlier your cravings start.

• Remove the sugar bowl from your life — you don't need it. Like salt, sugar is an acquired taste built up over years, so you need to eliminate it from your life slowly until the habit is at a level that is not causing you to crave it as much or put on weight from consuming it.

• Added sugar is in most packaged foods, so cut back the amount you buy; this alone will reduce your sugar intake.

Lazy Bottom Line

• Food comes in great, good, and not-so-good categories. But it's all okay, and can all be eaten as part of a normal, healthy diet. If any food or drink is over-consumed, it will likely make you fat and could make you unhealthy or unwell.

• You need to eat vegetables — they're a very important part of life. Aim for five servings a day.

• Two servings of fruit a day are fine, and if you're not overweight, more is great. However, remember you're trying to lose weight: Eating lots of fruit will not help, nor will eating lots of anything!

• Sugar and salt are part of a normal diet. However, 90% of us eat too much of both, and often we have no idea. Cut your packaged-food intake in half, and you'll more than likely cut these two things in half as well.

• Treat sugar and salt like habits you've got into over the years. Slowly decrease your consumption, the habit will go, and presto — you'll taste real food again!

• Red meat is good for us, but we eat too much of it. Two to three servings of beef, pork, lamb, veal, or kangaroo are fine, but try to find other alternatives on the other days (or have meat-free days).

• Alcohol is not bad; however, it is now listed by world health organisations as a cancer risk, so you need to weigh the pros and cons of drinking not just for weight loss, but for your general health and well-being.

• Drinking anything other than water or maybe unsweetened black or green tea and coffee will add to weight gain if you don't include them in your daily food intake. The best thing to do is avoid all flavoured or fizzy drinks. If you're drinking these on a daily basis, stop and review your consumption. If you can't go without them, delegate them to treat status — not hydration status.

Corn dextrin is a thickener often used in fast-food burgers. It's also used as glue for postage stamps and envelopes.

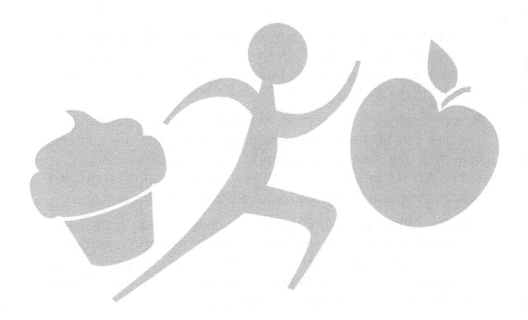

Chapter 12 – How Fit Are We?

Are you fit?

You wouldn't be alone if you said you didn't know. But how do you tell? And if you aren't fit, then how fit would you like to be?

Most people I talk to only want to be as fit as it takes to shed some weight or achieve a certain fitness goal like running a fun run or even a marathon. We don't tend to think of fitness as a lifelong thing that has to be worked on and maintained for life. However, we're not going to be losing weight or running marathons for life, but fitness levels need to be maintained for far more important reasons.

Exercise is not just about burning off calories; it's more than that. Exercise keeps our bodies going and us alive and well. It's also proven that it improves our quality of life, and will allow us to live longer — that is what we all want.

All forms of physical activity work our organs and muscles, especially our most important muscle: The heart. The more we pump oxygen-rich blood through it, the better it works, and the healthier it keeps us.

Moving keeps our bones strong. Weight-bearing exercise like walking and running builds strong bones, preventing the onset of diseases like osteoporosis and even osteoarthritis. The old adage "use it or lose it" applies.

Research is finding the benefits of exercise in our lives astounding. Exercise can help fight depression, can ward off many cancers, help with the healing of cancers, and keep some cancers in remission. The latest findings on how exercise can delay or even cure and improve the symptoms of dementia are amazing.

Exercise, physical activity, sport, or simply moving more helps everyone's quality of life, not just the overweight or obese. We all benefit: Young, old, fat, thin, fit, and unfit. New research shows that heavier people who exercise daily are fitter and live longer than skinny people who don't exercise.

Functional fitness

The new buzz phrase today in the fitness industry is functional fitness. It means the fitness and health activities we're doing are meaningless if they don't give us healthier, happier lifestyles and help us be disease-free and live longer. Exercise needs to be functional and relevant to our lives.

There was a time when people were either fit or unfit. How we defined the two was usually by the size of the person, the sport or fitness activity levels they had, and maybe whether they smoked. But now fitness has a range of definitions and meanings.

A barrage of tests can tell us exactly how fit or unfit we are. Blood tests show how healthy our body systems are, and body-composition testing tells us if we're in ideal weight ranges and if our body-fat, muscle-mass, and hydration ratios are okay. There are different fitness tests that show us if we have good cardio fitness, how strong we are, and how flexible we can be; we even have scans to see how fit our brains are! If we fail any of these tests, we are told what we need to do to improve that area of fitness.

Fat cells exist in all parts of the body except the eyelids, parts of the oesophagus, the brain, and the penis.

Fitness levels are personal, and individuals dictate how fit they want to be.

There have been times when I felt unfit after running a tough 10 km event, as I know I can run marathons. But many people who can't run to the letter box would think 10 km is an amazing distance to run. A parent's fitness goal could be to become fit enough to chase their kids around a park for an hour. Older people may want to stay fit so they can get through life's normal range of activities, like incorporating the right amount of cardio fitness to walk up the stairs at home or strength to open a jar of jam. It's all relevant to where you are and what you want to achieve with your fitness.

There are five categories of fitness, and although it seems like a lot, being aware of each level and knowing where you're at is a good thing.

1. Cardiovascular fitness

Cardiovascular refers to the heart (cardio) and blood vessels (vascular). The term is used in reference to how effectively the heart pumps blood and oxygen through the body. Cardio fitness is about working the heart and, in turn, pumping the blood. It's all the activities that work this system harder: Running, cycling, dancing, aerobics, etc.

To improve your cardio fitness, you need to get your heart pumping at a higher level and keep it there for an extended period of time: Approximately 45 minutes to an hour.

Other ways to improve cardio fitness are to take your heart rate through a range of levels. This can be achieved by doing short, fast spurts of speed interspersed by recovery activities, like walking then jogging and then walking again, or running then running faster. These sessions are called tempo or interval training.

It's easy to know if you are working your cardiovascular system: You should breathe faster and heavier, get sweaty, become red-faced, and feel uncomfortable.

Cardio-fitness activities reduce the risk of cardiovascular diseases and high blood pressure, and also help prevent osteoarthritis and osteoporosis. Cardio fitness is the best style of training for weight loss. If you're trying to lose weight, cardio fitness activities should be on the right side of your Lazy Loser scales on four to five occasions a week.

2. Muscular-strength fitness

This is when we do activities to build and strengthen our muscles or muscle groups. It usually means giving your muscles resistance (weight) and getting them to lift it or move it over several repetitions. After a few weeks of doing this resistance work, the muscle responds by growing and getting stronger. You then need to add more resistance to continue to grow the muscle and strengthen it.

Strength training is good for toning, and the stronger and bigger the muscles, the more calories they burn. Strength training doesn't mean you have to hit the gym and start weightlifting; it can come from any form of resistance. Walking or running up hills, exercises that use your own body as a resistance (push-ups, squats, lunges, etc.), and classes like yoga and Pilates can build strength.

3. Muscular-endurance fitness

This sounds similar to muscular-strength fitness, but it's different. This training is when your muscles are resisting continually for a long time, so you're building muscle as well as endurance. The muscles are strengthened in a different way, and it often builds a leaner muscle.

Muscular-endurance activities include cross-country running (where there's lots of resistance while you're running), long-distance running or walking, cycling, or skiing (one to two hours). The muscles are always working to keep you upright and still moving. Other activities in this category are boxing (where the arms are held high for a long period of time), rowing machines, and steppers for longer periods of time.

Muscular-endurance fitness is effective for reducing the risk of cardiovascular disease, diabetes, and obesity-related conditions.

4. Flexibility

I know we often cringe when we hear this word (well, someone like me who is very un-bendy does!). However, flexibility doesn't just mean being able to touch your toes or wrap your legs around your head.

Flexibility refers to being able to go through daily life, moving freely without pain. Ideally, we want every joint in our body to perform the FROM (Full Range of Movement), and flexibility allows that. We want to be able to get in and out of the car without pain, go up and down steps, and get out of bed easily.

If you have trouble doing those things or experience pain doing them, then it's time to work on your flexibility. Stretching after sporting activities, yoga, Pilates, or exercising in the water are all good at improving flexibility.

5. Body composition

You're probably thinking, If I do the four types of exercises above, then I shouldn't have to worry about this one — it will be ok after all that exercise. Sorry, but this is not always true. Body composition refers to everything inside of you.

Our bodies are made up of bone, muscle, blood (and fluids), and yes, fat as well. Fat is vital: Low body fat can be as unhealthy as high body fat. We need to be in the recommended range, and luckily all the above fitness activities help keep us there.

However, it's still true that we are what we eat. High-fat foods, greasy takeaways, and lots of sugar and alcohol are not good for our body compositions. Not all fat people drop dead of heart attacks, or have high cholesterol or high blood pressure and diabetes. I know lots of active, fit people who suffer from some of those diseases.

This is why it's important to have annual health checks. Go to the doctor, get your blood pressure checked, and make sure you know what your cholesterol levels are.

> Most people gain an average of just 1 g of extra body fat a day; 1 g a day equals 365 g of extra body fat a year. A gain of 365 g every year after the age of 25 would mean that by the time you hit your 50th birthday, you'd have laid down an extra 9 kilos (20 lb.) of excess body fat – or, as it's better known, middle-aged spread!

The Lazy way to exercise

Now you're thinking about how to fit all of the above in. It's no good being fit and healthy physically, then dropping dead of stress and exhaustion!

First, you need to like what you do. I'm always repeating this mantra: You will not do what you don't like for very long, so the No. 1 thing should be finding an activity you like to do rather than one you feel you should be doing.

However, don't automatically discount any activity you did years ago (like at school) and hated; things change, but more importantly, you've changed since then. So give it another go — take it slowly, build up your distances and intensity, and you may find you really enjoy something you thought you always hated.

There are hundreds of sports and exercises you can get involved in. Knowing what suits you, your timetable, and your budget can be hard. I suggest to any newbie exercisers or people who haven't exercised for a long time to get (back) into it slowly.

Don't base your exercise regime on the short term; your fitness should be for life. It's fine to join a gym, sign up for a new sport, or go to boot-camp or fitness classes, but make sure it's backed up with things you can do yourself. Pick an activity you can do anywhere at any time (e.g., walking, running, cycling, swimming), so you'll have a backup exercise. Then when the tennis, netball, cricket and footy seasons end, or boot-camp class finishes, you'll still know how to get out and exercise in between.

Lazy Bottom Line

- Fitness is an individual thing, but we need to include some form of exercise and fitness or activity into our lives.

- Cardio fitness burns energy from the food you eat: The more you do and the harder you work, the more calories you'll burn.

- Strength training builds muscles: The bigger the muscles, the more heat they use, and the more calories they burn as well.

- Flexibility is an important part of fitness. It's no good being able to run 10 km and then not be able to get out of bed or walk up and down the stairs without pain!

- Fitness isn't only for aesthetics. Visceral fat (fat on the inside) is from eating crap, and no amount of exercise will remove it — you still need to adjust your diet.

- Spread the fitness elements over your week. It will keep you from getting bored, and give a better overall feeling of health and well being.

- Do what you like! If you hate going to the gym, stop going. If you like walking, walk — you can try walking faster or insert some hills, stairs, or the beach into your walking course. If you enjoy your activity, it won't feel like exercise.

If spot reduction worked, all gum chewers would have skinny faces!

Chapter 13 – Excusercise

Excusercise (n.) — The (ir)rational psychological, sociological, physiological, environmental, or spiritual barriers/reasons/excuses individuals employ to avoid participation in unstructured physical activity or structured exercise.

I had to put this chapter in next, as I knew while you were reading the last chapter you were also thinking up an excuse as to how you can't exercise regularly. So, as usual, I'm one step ahead of you.

The reasons people don't exercise are many and varied, but they're all just excuses! Here are the top exercise excuses and my usual comebacks:

1. I don't have enough time.

Let's do the math: 168 hours in a week equates to...

• 56 hours of sleep. You want more, you say? I'll give you an extra hour a night, so change that to 63 hours.

• 40 hours of paid work ("MORE!" you yell at me? 50 hours it is).

• Half an hour per meal, which is 10.5 hours a week.

• Now you're asking, "What about getting to work or school or dropping off kids?" I'll allow another hour a day for travel incidentals, so seven hours.

• "What about 'me' time, social time, or just sitting-like-a-blob time?" No worries: Blob time is one hour a day, equating to a total of seven hours.

GRAND TOTAL = 137.5 hours

There are still 30.5 hours left over in your week. If you exercise for seven hours a week, that still leaves 23.5 hours for what? Maybe more blob time, sleep time, or even more exercise; it's up to you how to use those hours.

No-time tips

Write your seven hours of exercise time in your diary over the week. If it's written in like an appointment, you'll do it. Cross each off as you've done it. If it's not crossed off, it doesn't go away; add another 15 minutes on to four days that week, and you're all caught up!

Multi-task: Try to combine your exercise with something else you have to do. Can you walk, ride a bike, or run to work? Remember, I gave you time for that, so double-dip and use it for exercise.

Do you have to run kids around after school to sports or lessons? Don't just sit in the car, wait, or visit the supermarket. Wear your sports gear and while they're having their lesson, go for a run or walk. If it's swimming lessons, you jump in and swim as well.

2. I hate exercise!

Oh that's a pity, because everyone else loves it! We jump out of bed each morning bright and bouncy and love to get hot, out of breath, sweaty and smelly! Can you sense any sarcasm here?

I've been running for 25 years. Do I love it? No, not all the time — some days I hate getting up and putting my running shoes on, and some days it's okay, but no, I don't love it. I do it because it suits me; it fits in with my lifestyle and keeps me fit. If you ask any of my running buddies, they'll tell you I'm the biggest whinger of the lot when I'm running with them.

Fitness-marketing hype showing super fit and overly cheerful, enthusiastic personal trainers telling us how much fun it is sends the wrong message. It makes the rest of us think, *Oh, I'm not enjoying it, so I mustn't be doing it right or I'm not good at it.* Like many things in life, some days we like it, some days not, and other times we just do it because we have to.

Tips for the exercise hater

You do not have to love exercise; don't give up just because you think you're not enjoying it. It can be hard and it's supposed to be, but tell yourself the harder you work, the more health benefits you'll reap.

More often, it's the thought of getting up and out the door that's the problem; once you're there, you're fine, and often happy you made the effort. Remember that, when you're grumbling to yourself as you're getting ready to go.

You don't have to love exercise, but liking it is good, and you'll feel a sense of achievement when it's over. After a while, you'll start to see improvements in your body and health. Those are the things you'll like and appreciate — not the actual exercise.

There are so many exercise styles and sports out there to try; I'm sure there's one that you feel is okay, that you can do and that suits you. Don't be waiting for light bulbs and euphoric moments; just tell yourself, "Okay, I can manage this . . . it suits me, and I think I can get better at it." That's all you need to know.

I suggest you give any new exercise three months. Commit to doing it three or four times a week, and set yourself a goal in that time. If it's running: 5 km without stopping; for walking: One hour, upping the intensity so you feel it working for you. For fitness classes, getting through a whole class without feeling like dying is a very good goal to have. If at the end of the three months, you gave it your all and didn't reach your goal, feel any great benefit, or still don't enjoy it, then you can say, "Okay, I gave it a good shake and it's not for me. I'm going to try something else."

Don't just take on something for a week; the first week is the worst! You need to see improvements and feel you're achieving something before you throw the towel in.

> If you can't pronounce one of the ingredients on the food label, don't buy it.

I like the high feeling when I've finished my run, I enjoy running events, and I love the reward coffee afterward. But I don't like running all the time, and often I find long training runs tiring and boring. But I keep my mind focused on the reasons I run.

Remember: It doesn't have to be the actual exercise that you enjoy — it's often the rewards and how you feel afterward.

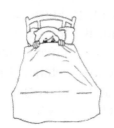

3. I can't get out of bed!

I don't know how to break this to you, but you can get out of bed — you do it on a daily basis, so I know you can.

How do you get up if you have to get to the airport, go to work, or get to an appointment? You set an alarm, and when it goes off, you get up and go about your business. So why can't you do the same thing with exercise? Just get up!

Make a deal with yourself: Three mornings a week, you're going to get up an hour earlier to exercise. That leaves four mornings a week to not get up. Come on, you can't be fairer than that! You can stay in bed more than you have to get up. On weekends, you can exercise anytime, so no alarms.

Tips for the bed-hugger

I suggest if you're not an enthusiastic exerciser that you try to get it done in the morning, as you'll find a lot more excuses not to exercise as the day drags on. The only thing going on between 6 and 7 a.m. in your life is probably sleep, so take that hour and convert it to exercise. If you like 8 or 9 hours of sleep a night, that's fine and normal; I'm not telling you to go without sleep. On the three mornings you've allocated to early exercise, go to bed an hour earlier the night before. Problem solved!

It's all about making deals with yourself and setting schedules; it will not happen without planning and preparation.

4. I look silly and feel stupid.

Here's something to think about: When you're running or in a gym class or any other exercise group, do you think all the other people out on the street and in the gym are looking at you? I hate to burst your bubble, but I don't even think they know you're in the room or have even noticed you on the street.

I know that's true. When I'm running, I couldn't even tell you who or what I saw or how I felt about them. I'm so busy trying to keep myself going that I have no idea who is looking stupid or silly out there besides myself.

I've been running and around runners long enough to know we're all happy to see other runners out there getting fit. It's the same in gyms with all of those scary mirrors; have a look in the mirror and check out what the others are looking at. They're either watching the gym instructor, looking at themselves, or looking at gorgeous girls or hunky trainers. Sorry to disappoint, but they're not ogling you!

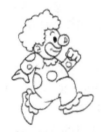

Tips for the silly looking

Wear clothing you feel comfortable and not overexposed in. You don't have to wear crop tops and bike pants to exercise; cover up in cool, light clothing that doesn't cling to all the curves and you don't feel you're hanging out of.

Try my trick: Wear a hat. You're always invisible when you have a hat on!

Start off in beginners' classes, where you know the others are just getting into the sport or activity as well and probably feel just as silly and stupid as you. Realise that those feelings are all in your head, and no one is interested in or looking at you. Sad but true.

Lazy Tale

I'm usually oblivious to all things when running — I'm deep inside my head, pushing myself, or enjoying the view. I'm also the pinup girl for the RUN UGLY campaign, as I'm usually sweating, snorting, and blowing like a water buffalo, so most people tend to look away from, rather than at, me!

Last year, my 17-year-old daughter, Rosemary, wanted to get back into running, and asked me to go for a run with her. We decided to run along the beautiful river in

Noosaville, which can be very busy in the evening with all forms of exercisers.

After about five minutes of running, I felt a few people looking at me when I ran past. I thought maybe I knew them, but realised I didn't; a bit further on, I noticed more looks in my direction. I started to stress — did I have bits and pieces hanging out? Was there a wardrobe malfunction with my sports bra? I looked down and checked, but saw all wiggly bits well covered and strapped in.

The looks, glances, and even smiles continued. I'd been chatting to Rosemary all the way, encouraging her to concentrate on good running technique: Head high, shoulders back and down, tall stance, etc.

About three quarters of the way through the run, people were still looking my way, and my paranoia was growing. I turned to Rose to ask if I had anything on my face, as people were staring at me. Then the penny dropped: I was running beside the new updated version of Bo Derek in the movie 10! Rosemary is a beautiful girl; she had on short shorts and a skimpy top, and there she was bounding and bouncing along effortlessly beside me.

Moral of the story is proof of my point above: No one is looking at you. Believe me, there are far nicer things to look at when you're running, so don't worry about looking silly!

5. Exercise is boring.

You got that right! I'm going to blame the highly excitable personal trainers and fitness fanatics again for the perception that we should be filled with boundless excitement when exercising. There's nothing more exciting than lifting a weight while the trainer counts slowly upward and then, oh, the highs of them counting downward slowly!

Exercise can be dull sometimes — there, I said it. However, what do you want from it? Endless stimulation thrills and spills every second? If so, maybe you should take up Formula One driving. If you want fitness and weight loss, be prepared for dull moments!

The reason I started running was that I had four small children, and I also worked. So often I would roll out of bed in the dark to go for a run for a few minutes of peace and alone time. I was craving dull and boring!

What's wrong with being bored? We seem to live in a society that thinks boredom is a dirty word, and every second needs to be fulfilling and exciting.

Tips for the bored

Once again, you need to work it your way, if you're out running or walking, take the chance to have some good quality think time. If you love music, lose yourself and listen to the music you want to listen to. Don't think "boring"; think, "Ahhh, peace!"

However, if that doesn't work, stop it from being boring! Find a running buddy, chat, gossip, bitch, whatever — you'll be amazed how quickly the time flies.

Play a sport for exercise — that is never boring. I played tennis in a small mothers'-group competition for years, and it was great fun. We worked hard when we were on the court, but also had lots of laughs and once again, the coffee at the end was the best bit.

Team sports require working together and focusing on a goal. Don't tell me you could ever get bored doing that — you don't get time to think of anything else but exactly what you're doing in the moment.

Try mixing up your activities to stop the boredom or monotony, but that doesn't mean you should drop the boring stuff altogether. Things like running, walking, rowing, swimming laps, or cycling for miles could be classed as boring, but they can also be the things that bring you peace and satisfaction, and allow you to work at your own pace.

Then there are activities like surfing and skiing that require so much concentration you don't have time to think about anything

Calorie/kilojoule conversion: Approximately four kilojoules equal one calorie.

Lazy Loser

else except staying upright and moving forward. All the above types of activities can be covered during your week; the change in activity, pace, and workout is enough to get rid of any boredom.

6. It's too expensive.

It can be, but it doesn't have to be. A gym membership can cost between $500 and $1,000 a year, but remember, if you go three or four times a week, that's not so expensive. And don't get me started on golf fees or the cost of a road bike.

However, I'm not going to let you use the money excuse, as there are many things you can do for zilch. Running, walking, swimming (if you have your own pool or can go to the beach or river), and cycling are all free.

Tips for the penny saver

You do not need expensive equipment to exercise. For running you should have a good pair of running shoes — that's vital, and will cost anywhere from $80 to $200, but that's it. An old T-shirt and shorts are sufficient for the rest. You don't need a racing bike to cycle, but if you do want to go that way, there are plenty of second-hand ones out there to get you started. I bet someone you know has a good bike in his or her shed that they'd love you to borrow for a while. And as for swimming — lash out on a pair of goggles! Walking is free and you can wear whatever is in your wardrobe.

There are many council fitness programs that are free or cost next to nothing. They often have walking groups, running clubs, tai chi, and yoga or outdoor exercise classes; all you need to do is make a phone call to find out more.

You don't have to join a gym either, most parks in cities and towns have exercise equipment and instructions on how to use them, it's your free outdoor gym.

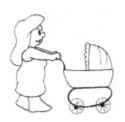

7. I have small children, and can't get away.

I hear you, and as I said above, the only reason I started running was so I could get it over and done with early to be home before my little darlings woke up. You may need to accept that this is what you have to do for fitness for a few years (or in my case, about 15!). Set your alarm and get up and going before they know you're gone.

There are many ways to stay fit with your kids. I remember riding around town for hours with a toddler in the seat on the back of my bike. He loved it, and I was getting my exercise in — win/win.

Then along came number two. That was harder, so I went to the double pram and I'd walk around town for hours! It was hard work: Both strength and cardio fitness.

Tips for the tied down

It's normal to want to exercise without screaming kids in tow. Most gyms and swimming pools have crèches — use them. You get a workout in, and the kids have fun.

But here's the best tip: Ask someone for help (you're allowed to do that you know)! You only need an hour, and I'm sure there are lots of people (family, friends or neighbours) who wouldn't mind taking the kids for that time.

Get a few friends together in a babysitting circle, where one has the kids once a week while the other parents go off and exercise, and you swap it around so everyone gets a chance to work out kid free. I'm sure lots of your friends with little ones would love that idea, and if it were me, I wouldn't be thinking of the exercise — I'd be thinking of the great social coffee afterward. Another win/win!

I'm going to leave it there. I know there are many more excuses, and maybe there's a book in me called "Lazy Excuses". But remember, they're just that: Excuses. All can be dealt with, overcome, and sorted. Stop excusercising and get moving.

Lazy Bottom Line

• Making time to exercise sounds hard, but when you sit down and work out your weekly timetable, you'll find the time to fit it in.

• Make appointments with yourself to exercise. Cancel that appointment, and you have to reschedule within 24 hours of cancellation.

- You don't have to love exercise. Go with the basics: You like it sometimes, and you can do it. If you love it, that's a bonus, but you won't be alone if you don't!

- If you have trouble getting out of bed to exercise, set the alarm!

- No one is looking or laughing at you when you're exercising. Most people are just like you: Trying to get from A to B and live to tell the story.

- Want to be invisible out there? Wear a cap.

- Exercise can be boring! Get used to it. Think of it more as peace and quiet.

- It doesn't have to cost an arm and a leg to exercise. There are plenty of things to do that cost nothing, like walking, swimming, and running.

Chapter 14 – Don't Exercise, Then!

In the last two chapters, I've tried hard to make you see how wonderful exercise can be for you and your long-term health. I've talked about how great it is for speeding up weight loss, and how to get into it easily.

However, if after all that blabbing on you're still determined that you are not going to exercise — then don't!

Often it's the term "exercise" or "sport" that makes us think, *Oh that's hard,* or *That's boring,* or *I'm not into that.*

Exercise and sport make many couch potatoes think of commando-style boot camps; gyms full of muscle-bound youths ogling themselves in the mirror; competitive sports on TV where every five minutes someone is being carted off on a stretcher; or the best athletes in the world standing on a dais and getting a medal placed around their necks. And, of course, we don't see or want to see ourselves in any of those scenarios.

If that's what you think exercise is, then don't exercise! What if I told you that you never have to do it, or say it, or think it . . . would that make you happy?

Good. You never have to exercise — ever.

But maybe you can do this: Move. Just get up and do something. No, you don't have to go anywhere, join anything, or buy new fancy gear; just get out and about. Have fun doing something outdoors — play, dance, wrestle the kids or the dog — anything.

If you hate exercise, below are some things you can do. No, they're not going to hurt or turn you into that buff stud you don't want to be, and they have nothing to do with improving your health or losing weight, so don't panic.

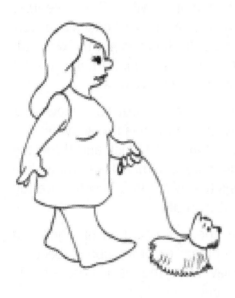

1. Walk your dog. No, it's not for you — it's for the benefit of your poor pooch and your responsibility as a pet owner.

2. Show your baby the world, in his or her pram. It's not exercise — it's your responsibility as a proud parent!

3. Teach your children how to ride a bike. It's not for your benefit, but you don't want them to go through life never knowing how. This means you have to run or walk along beside them so they don't crash, or ride along with them so they don't get hit by a car. It's your job to be a good parent.

4. Take a holiday! There's no exercise in that statement. Ride your bike (or walk or run) to work to save on public transport or petrol. You could save $50 to $100 a week, then go and lie on a beach somewhere for a 10 days once a year and do absolutely nothing. That's not exercising — it's giving you a well-deserved break.

5. Save the planet. Walking to the shops has nothing to do with your health; you are an environmentalist, and this is your way of getting one carbon-eater off the street.

6. Find a cure for a deadly disease or help starving children. Enter a charity fun run, walk, or cycle that supports a worthwhile cause.

Naturally, you'll need to train and get fitter, but it's not for your benefit — it's to save the lives of thousands.

7. Be community-spirited. Volunteer your services to your local national park, botanical gardens, or beaches — they're always looking for volunteers to clean up these areas. Mow someone else's lawn; there are many elderly people who require this service.

8. Have a gossip. Now, who doesn't like this type of activity? I had a great friend who lived around the corner from me for years. Three times a week, we would txt each other with, "Got some juicy news." We'd meet at a halfway point between our houses and walk for an hour, gossiping the whole way. Our tongues got the workout, and we never looked on it as exercise: It was just a catch-up. So don't gossip on the phone or at work — walk and talk.

9. Set an example. You may hate exercise, but you know your children need to understand how important healthy activities are in their lives, so it's up to you. Someone has to kick and throw the ball, run and hide, push the swing, chase, demonstrate trampoline tricks — all those wonderful things that teach kids how to have fun and stay fit (and I bet you'll love it as well).

10. Earn some extra money. Like the idea of a part-time job and a bit of extra cash? Deliver pamphlets or newspapers, become a professional dog walker, mow lawns on the weekends, etc. No exercise here — just good, hard work.

There are 10 things that aren't exercise or sport, but they still go in the right of your Lazy Loser scales.

All that's required of you is to do something active. Label it what you want, but it's good for your family, the community, and your pets. And if it improves your health or helps you lose weight, oh well — you'll just have to grin and bear it!

Fat cells die at the rate of 150 per second.

Lazy Bottom Line

• You don't have to do formal exercise to be fit and healthy.

• The best form of activity is what fits in with you and your lifestyle and makes you feel good.

• Stop turning exercise into a chore. If you don't like what you're doing for your fitness, find something you do like.

• All movement helps, so work on getting more of it into your day.

• If solo activities bore you, recruit company — the kids, your dog, a mate, etc.

• Get an active job! Earn money and get fit: a great combination.

A person is considered obese when his or her weight is 20% or more above the normal weight.

Chapter 15 – Lazy Gym

When I first coined the phrase Lazy Runner several years ago, many people laughed at the oxymoron; how could those two words be linked? It's a bit like "fun" and "run"!

Lazy Runner was referring to me. Sure I ran and could run a long way if I wanted to, but I always approached running from a fun, healthy perspective. My theory was, "I'm not very good at other sports and activities, but I can run. I enjoy it (most of the time), and it keeps me at a healthy weight range and fit." Running suited me, 25 years later it is still doing those things, and now, of course, it's my healthy habit. I soon found there were lots of Lazy Runners out there like me.

So when I say Lazy Gym, I'm using the same analogy. Chapter 12 tells you all about the types of fitness, and how we need to implement them — not just in the short term, but for life. I've taught hundreds of people how to run, and also how to enjoy running. Half of them had never run a step in their lives and spent much of their first meeting with me telling me why they couldn't run. Once I taught them the Lazy way, they were hooked, and had a great fitness skill for life.

Lazy Loser

Many people, especially overweight ones, are fearful of starting any new fitness routine. They feel fat, silly, or scared they won't be able to do it, or that they'll make a fool of themselves or get injured. The thought of joining a boot camp or gym scares the hell out of them. All these thoughts and fears are relevant, but they won't get you moving.

One way to cope with the stress and fear of exercise is to take charge and do it yourself. I've devised a DIY fitness regime that I call Lazy Gym. You don't have to sign up or pay one cent to join Lazy Gym: Put on some comfy gear and walk out your front door. Welcome to your own Lazy Gym!

Here are a few things you need to know about getting fit:

1. You don't need to join a gym.

2. You don't need to suffer through a six-week boot-camp program and not be able to get out of bed without pain for those six weeks.

3. You don't need a personal trainer.

4. You don't need to buy expensive gym equipment.

However, if you like the idea of trying any of those things, then go for it. But if money is an issue for you; finding the time to get to these programs is too hard and stressful; or you're worried about the intensity and pain of joining an exercise program, then don't do it. There are so many other things you can do to get fitter. Reread chapter 14 to get some ideas.

But you do want to exercise, don't you? You just have no idea of how to go about it. Lazy Gym will show you how.

The programs below cover all fitness levels. If you've never exercised or haven't for many years, start with the Lazy Walking Program or Lazy Gym Circuit Program.

Fat-free does not mean calorie-free; too many calories from sugars and starches add extra weight, too.

Lazy Walking Program

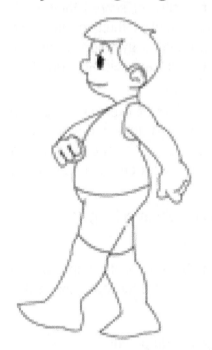

If you've never exercised or haven't in a long time, go to your doctor and tell him or her what you plan to do. Take this book and show them the program you intend to start on. He/she will give you a check over and let you know if it's a suitable program for your level of health and fitness.

To start, walk straight out your front door and up the street. Keep walking for 20 minutes, remember the landmark you get to, and turn and walk back. All done!

Now you need to assess your walk. Was it easy? Did you start to sweat? Was it really tough?

If you found it hard, that's great — repeat the same walk tomorrow and for the rest of the week. It will get easier the more you do it.

If you found it easy and didn't work up a sweat, walk faster tomorrow and get to your turn landmark in 19.5 minutes. When you've finished, assess this walk. Still easy? The next day, get to the landmark in 19 minutes (run the last bit if you have to). Keep doing this until you get to your landmark in 17 minutes — that is fast walking.

Now it's time to increase your distance. This time, walk out 30 minutes, remember your landmark, and turn and walk back. Then it's back to speeding up again: The next day, get to the landmark in 29.5 minutes and continue your countdown of covering the same distance in a faster time.

Most fat-free and reduced-fat foods contain more sodium than their regular versions. Extra salt makes up for the flavour loss when manufacturers cut the fat.

Assess your walk every day. If it's starting to get easy, up the ante again with some speed or extra distance.

Do this type of walking five days a week. Then, on one day of the week, extend yourself.

Do one long walk lasting over an hour and a half. Make it interesting: Walk on parts of a beach, add in some hills or stairs, or do a bush walk. Don't worry about speed — this walk is designed to build some strength and endurance, so just walk and enjoy.

That's six days. On the seventh day, do you rest? No; it's fine to exercise daily. Your body will adapt better, and you'll see improvements much more quickly. Make the seventh day something very different — a yoga or Pilates class, swim, surf, cycle, ski — anything that uses different muscle groups and challenges you in other ways.

So there you have it: All your fitness needs sorted.

When you increase your speed, you work your cardio fitness; the long walk is good for endurance fitness; the hills, stairs, beach, or bush are good strength training; and one other different activity is ideal for using the other muscles groups that walking doesn't use. And if you stretch after each session or throw in a yoga class, you cover flexibility.

Lazy Runner Beginners' Program

Want to up the intensity?

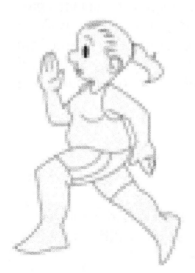

If you've been walking for a while and are bored or feel you're not pushing yourself as hard as you'd like, why not up the ante and start running? To find out all about getting into running, you need to buy my last book, "Lazy Runner". It has a whole chapter on beginner running, but here are a few beginner rules to get you started.

• Start running on an easy course — don't go out too far or run cross country, hills, or on the beach. Your first running course should be safe, flat, and easy.

• Map your course for 5 km: 2.5 km out and 2.5 km back. Now don't die of shock: You're not expected to run 5 km on day one. However, it's best to work on your 5 km course until you can run the whole way. 5 km running or walking is an ideal distance to be exercising for cardio fitness. You'll run/walk your course until the walks decrease and runs increase. It could take anywhere from six weeks to three months to run all the way; that's normal, so don't rush it.

• Start off running slowly (as slowly as you can). Most beginners run too fast, then get puffed very quickly.

• Don't stop the first time you feel like stopping; instead, pick a landmark (tree, road, or house) and run to that. Don't stop the second time you feel like stopping, either — find another landmark to run to. The third time you want to stop, walk for one minute. This system helps you push through the mental barrier and run farther. If you always stop the first time you want to, you'll never extend your running times. Remember: Push through twice and on the third time, stop running, but keep moving by walking, until you're fine to run again.

• When you do need to walk, keep an eye on how long you walk for. If you have a watch on, time your walk; one minute is enough. If you don't have a watch, count to 100, then start running again — slowly. Never walk for more time than you run. If you walk for longer than a minute, you lose all the great cardio build-up from the run section. You'll never run the distance you want to run if you walk too much. One minute is plenty of time to get your breath back.

We're eating out more: 35% of our weekly caloric intake is consumed in restaurants. That's up from 23% in the 1970s.

• Don't worry about running out of breath — it won't happen, and on the extremely rare occasions that it does, you'll be dead and won't have a worry in the world! If you feel you're losing your breath, try blowing all the air out of your lungs in three long, slow exhales, then start breathing normally again (don't stop running whilst you do this). A lot of the time, the running-out-of-breath feeling is panic. Use diversion techniques to get past this: Listen to music, enjoy the view, take a buddy with you. These things will make you stop stressing about your breathing.

• Don't start off running every day; every other day is enough. Running is new to your body, and 48 hours' rest in between is an ideal time for your body to recover. However, you can still walk on the non-run days to keep your fitness up.

• Be extra aware of your diet and fluid intake. Running can be intense and burns more energy, causing you to work harder and sweat more. You'll need more carbohydrates and fluids when you're a runner.

Once you get to be a runner — which means you can run 5 km without stopping and feel okay — then it's up to you what you do with your running. Like walking, you can opt to increase your speed. Run your 5 km 10 seconds faster each time until you're running the time you want to run it in. Or you can increase your distance: If you'd like to aim for 10 km, make one run a week half a kilometre longer.

Your 10 km training program could go like this:

Week 1: 2 x 5 km and 1 x 5.5 km

Week 2: 2 x 5 km and 1 x 6 km

Week 3: 2 x 5 km and 1 x 6.5 km

Week 4: 1 x 5 km, 1 x 6 km, and 1 x 7 km

Week 5: 1 x 5 km, 1 x 6 km and 1 x 7.5 km

Week 6: 1 x 5 km, 1 x 6 km and 1 x 8 km

Week 7: 1 x 5 km, 1 x 7 km and 1 x 8.5 km

Week 8: 1 x 5 km, 1 x 8 km and 1 x 9 km

Week 9: 1 x 5 km, 1 x 7 km and 1 x 9.5 km

Week 10: 1 x 5 km, 1 x 8 km and 1 x 10 km

As you can see, it takes time to get to 10 km, and this is the safest way to do it. Upping the distances too quickly can lead to injury. Always leave the shorter distances in your running week; they'll start to become easy, and you'll enjoy them more. You may even like to lift the pace on the shorter runs, which will increase your cardio fitness.

Then what? Enter a 10 km fun run!

Final points about the Lazy Walking and Running programs:

1. Set the time or distance you're going to walk or run and get out and do it. 5 km or 45 minutes is an ideal distance and time to walk or run for fitness. When it gets easier, go faster or longer.

2. Walk or run from your home; it's more time efficient. However, if you live in an area that doesn't have safe walking paths, isn't scenic, or has lots of hills, drive to a nicer, scenic, safe, flat area, and walk or run there.

3. Treadmill running and walking are good alternatives if the weather is bad, it's dark, or you feel unsafe outdoors. Follow the same programs outlined above. I do recommend running or walking outside at least once a week. It will give you more confidence, and prevents boredom that can come with exercising indoors.

4. Running and brisk walking burns energy, and that can make you sweat more. Not replacing those fluids can make you feel fatigued, headachy, or even nauseous, so make sure you increase your fluid intake (just drink more water).

Lazy Gym Circuit Program

Walking and running are great, but they can get boring, and then you lose your motivation to get yourself out there each day. These two activities are good weight-bearing exercises to improve your cardio fitness; however, if you want to get fitter, stronger, and make your workouts more interesting, you can do circuit training.

Find an area that suits your Lazy Gym Circuit; hopefully you have a park or beach or playground near where you live. Often at these places, you will find a covered area, paths, steps, hills, benches, etc. All of these things are great for your Lazy Gym.

Speed circuits

These are suitable for runners and walkers and are a good way to get faster and burn more calories.

Measure out a 1 km loop at your park or beach area. If you can't find a 1 km distance, go for 500 m (half a km). The reason 1 km is ideal is because it takes five loops to run or walk 5 km, and as I mentioned above, 5 km is a good distance to work on.

Make your start point near a drink tap, or take your drink bottle and hide it under a tree or bench so you can get water after each loop.

Below are a few speed-circuit variations you can do:

1. Warm up by walking or running a loop and time it. 2nd loop: Walk or run 10 seconds faster; 3rd Loop: Walk or run 10 seconds faster than loop 2; 4th Loop: Walk or run 10 seconds faster than loop 3; 5th Loop: Walk or run it as fast as you can. Grab your drink, walk until you've cooled down, then stretch.

2. Warm up by walking or slow running a loop. 2nd Loop: Walkers do a slow jog, runners run as fast as you can; 3rd loop: Recovery jog for runners, walkers just walk; 4th Loop: Walkers do a slow jog; runners run as fast as you can; 5th Loop: Recovery jog for runners and walkers just walk. Stretch.

3. Short tempo running or walking. Break loops into sections (it could be light poles or trees). 1st Loop: Warm up by jogging or walking; 2nd Loop: Walkers alternate fast and slow walking between your short landmarks, runners jog and run fast between short landmarks; 3rd Loop: Walk or run normally; 4th Loop: Walkers alternate fast and slow walking between your short landmarks, runners jog and run fast between short landmarks; 5th Loop: Cool-down jog or walk; stretch.

Fidgeters — You're not likely to see a fat fidgeter. Those people who twiddle their thumbs, wriggle in their seats, and jump up down continually to go and get things burn up to 380 calories or more than the calm, non-fidgeters.

Stop in between each loop and have a drink or two minutes of rest. On the speed portion of each section, you should be working hard — puffing, sweating, hot and even bothered. These are signs that you're working your cardiovascular system.

Cardio and strength Lazy circuits

Now you have the running and walking circuits sorted, you can add in some strength work. Many towns have gym areas in parks with instructions on how to use the equipment. These are great — use them.

If you have outdoor fitness equipment in your area, use it for your circuit training.

Once again, map out a walk or run loop near the equipment of approximately 500 m to 1 km.

Start with a warm-up walk or jog, then use the exercise equipment. Make sure you read the directions first, so you know you're doing it properly. Do five repetitions on each piece of equipment, then run/walk your loop again. Next, do 10 repetitions on each, then walk/run your loop again. For your last set of repetitions, do 15 on each piece, then set off for a final cool-down run/walk.

Assess how you feel after this session. Was it easy? Did you feel it burning? It's best to wait for 24 hours to see how your muscle groups feel the next day. If you feel like a truck ran over you in the night, that's OK — it's your muscles telling you they're fatigued and will be ready to repeat the same circuit in 48 hours. However, if you feel good and have no sore bits, up the ante.

On your next session, keep the walk/run loops, but increase your repetitions on the exercise equipment: Do 10 repetitions on the first set, 15 on the second, and 20 on the third. 24 hours later, assess this workout. Still feel good? Increase the repetitions again.

Keep working out this way. Do a circuit, assess it the next day, then either repeat the last session or increase the repetitions on the exercise equipment or the speed on the walk/run section.

Create your own Lazy Gym

Go to your local park, playground, or foreshore. Find an area that is suitable for you to work on. Use a park table, chairs, or bench; this will be your base. Walk a loop of the park first; hopefully that loop will be 500 m to 1 km, which is a great warm up. When you get back to your base, do these exercises:

1. Push-ups, abdominal crunches, triceps dips, side bends, squats, and step-ups (five each).

2. Walk or run your loop, then back to base.

3. Push-ups, abdominal crunches, triceps dips, side bends, squats, and step-ups (10 each).

4. Walk or run your loop, then back to base.

5. Push-ups, abdominal crunches, triceps dips, side bends, squats, and step-ups (15 each).

6. Get into the plank position and hold for 30 seconds.

7. Cool-down walk/jog the last loop, then go back to base.

8. Stretch and have a drink.

This session should take at least 45 minutes. Assess how you feel the day after. If you feel no exercise side effects, next time increase the exercise repetitions by five each-: That's 10 after the first loop, 15 after the second loop, and 20 after the third loop. With the plank, aim to hold it for an extra 10 seconds each time you do it (so 40 seconds).

Assess this workout. If you feel this one in some or all of your muscle groups, then stick with it for a week or two before upping the repetitions again.

The assessment is an important way to know whether a workout is working for you or whether it's not active enough. You don't want

Overweight people underestimate the size of their meals and the amount they eat by 40%; people of a healthy weight over estimate by 20%, meaning we all overestimate how much food we eat.

to be in pain after any session, but you should feel some fatigue in the muscles groups you've worked.

- Walking fast or running: General fatigue in legs
- Push-ups: Chest and arms
- Abdominal crunches: Tummy (upper, lower, and sides)
- Triceps dips: Back of upper arms
- Side bends: Muffin-top area
- Squats: Top of legs (quads) and bum
- Step-ups: Bum

You may feel tightness in some areas and nothing in others; this is when you need to adapt your repetitions. Push-ups can be tough — you're lifting your whole body or upper body off the ground — so you may find it hard to get to 10, whereas you may find the 10 triceps dips too easy. Increase the numbers on the exercises you don't feel (so, in the previous example, double your triceps dips), and keep the ones you do feel the same until they get to a point where you're ready to up the repetitions.

Bottom line: Don't do something that is too easy or too hard. There's a line between these two, and you need to find it and move on a continuum so you're getting the most out of your workouts.

Do your circuits three or four times a week. On the days you're not Lazy Gyming, be active in other ways. This doesn't even need to be exercise, as you can find lots of non-exercise activities in the last chapter (Chapter 14: Don't Exercise, Then!).

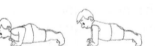

Squats

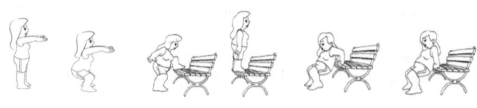

Step Ups

Tricep Dips

Push ups

The Plank

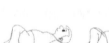

Crunches

Other Lazy Workouts

If you live near a beach, hit it. Most beaches have dunes, stairs, dry sand, wet sand, and of course, wonderful water: Perfect Lazy Gym conditions.

Try this on a beach:

• Walk up the sand hills and run down them for 10 minutes.

• Walk in the soft sand up the beach and run back on the hard sand near the water's edge for 10 minutes.

• Do a combination of backward walking or running (great for leg strength, and it doesn't matter if you fall on your bum in the sand), side steps, and lunges in the soft sand up the beach for 100 m. Walk or run back on the hard sand. Repeat for 10 minutes.

• Walk up and down the steps, if any, for 10 minutes.

• Get in the ocean until the water is over your knees and below your hips and walk strongly. Use big leg and arm movements and follow the shoreline. Do this for 10 minutes.

• Swim after your beach session for 10 to 20 minutes.

You can do a combination of all these things or just three of them. You have a great exercise routine, and it's all free!

Sand and water act as resistance. Imagine that they try to hold you back each step and you have to push through them. This takes strength, and it's all good fun.

Ride to your Lazy Workout

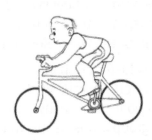

If you're not keen on the running and walking sections, replace them with riding your bike. Ride to a park, do your exercise repeats as outlined above, then jump on the bike and ride to another park and do them there. Keep it up until you get home (so maybe three bike rides at 10 minutes each and three park workouts).

Be your own Lazy Trainer

Your partner, kids, or a friend may like to join your Lazy Gym — sign them up!

On one session, you be the personal trainer: You call the shots, choose the exercises and repetitions, do the counting up and down, and give all the positive reinforcement (of course, you're doing the workout as well, not just standing there yelling like a sergeant major). On the next workout, they are the personal trainer, and you have to do the session they set for you. One day you're in charge, and the next day you're the victim (I mean client). This is fun, motivational, and never boring.

Lazy Swimming

This is a funny one for me to be writing about, as I can't swim! It is on my bucket list to learn how, but as of yet I haven't got around to it. However, I do know how great swimming can be for cardio and strength fitness. If you like to swim and or you have past injuries that prevent you from doing weight bearing exercises, swimming can be a good alternative.

If you can swim great; but if you are a non-swimmer or would like to be a better swimmer, have some lessons first. There are many adult learn to swim or technique correction lessons you can join at most aquatic centres. Running and walking are mostly no brainer activities, but with swimming you should be doing it right to get the best effects.

Allow 45-60 minutes for your swimming activity. Like all exercise you will start with some warm up laps, depending on how swim fit you are, you may need to start swimming a lap and then walking a lap and continue this until you are swimming for the whole session.

Then you can mix it up a bit. Swim your laps faster or change your swimming stroke each lap, so you get a variety in your workout. If you are getting bored swimming laps on your own, many pools have swim squads where you can swim in groups; this keeps your motivation going and improves your swimming as well.

Lazy Bottom Line

• Gyms, personal trainers, fitness classes, and boot camps are great; however, you don't need to sign up for anything or pay money to get fit.

• Allot 45 minutes to an hour a day to doing more. This doesn't have to be in an exercise format, but it does have to involve action-based activities.

• Set yourself a fitness program. If it's walking, great! Running? Fantastic! Working out at the park or beach? Brilliant.

• Assess every workout you do. Is it too easy or you feel nothing afterwards? Increase the intensity. Can't get out of bed the next day? Continue with the basic workout until it becomes comfortable (this could take a few weeks), then up the ante again.

• Your workout shouldn't be too easy or too hard; there is a huge gap between those levels of difficulty.

• If you have any past or recurrent injuries, some of the exercises above may aggravate them. If you notice any sign of pain that doesn't feel like normal exercise pain, cease the exercise.

• If you haven't exercised in years, have health issues or past injuries that have prevented you from exercising, get the all clear from your doctor first.

• Get out and do something each day; however, do intense exercise only three or four days a week. On the other days, opt for lower-impact workouts like yoga, Pilates, swimming, or walking.

Head for the hills! Men living close to sea level are five times more likely to be obese compared to those living at 3,000 metres or more above sea level. For women, it's four times more. It's believed that the low oxygen levels higher up affect metabolism, and may play a part in the statistics.

Chapter 16 – Mental Fat

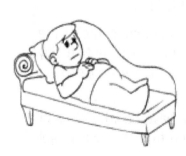

In my last publication, "Lazy Runner", I included a chapter on mental running. Now we have mental fat.

Most of what we achieve or don't achieve in life comes down to our mental attitude. When we're strong and focused mentally, we can do anything, but when we have self-doubt or feel insecure, it takes all our mental powers just to get us out of bed in the morning.

I've always lived by the premise, "Your body will do whatever you tell it to" — but you have to give it the right tools and directions. That's what your brain is for!

One litre of the water we consume in a day is from solid food.

Lazy Loser Mental Philosophy

1. Do you want to lose weight?

2. Is it high on your priority list?

3. Are you unhappy with your size, shape, and health and want to change them for the better?

If you answered "Yes" to any of the above and are still overweight and unhappy, then what the hell are you doing?

Are you still fat because you've tried and failed?

Then no more diets or health kicks for you.

Is it because you can't control your eating?

We know that's not right, as you do have control over what goes in your mouth.

Is it because you were a fat child and don't know how to change?

You're not a kid anymore — you are in charge, and you can change.

I think you can see where I'm going with this. It's good to know why you are overweight and have failed at losing weight in the past, but it's no good dwelling on it and using it as your lifetime excuse. It's time to move on.

Now you have no excuses: You admit that you're fat and can't lose weight.

That's better! But you can't seem to lose weight in the long term or keep it off. Now we have something real to work with.

Back to the original question: Do you really want to lose weight?

I believe if you really want to do something, you will and if you don't, you won't. It sounds simple, but if I look back to the things I've achieved in life and the things I've crashed and burned at (and yes, there have been plenty of these), I know that success has come if I've wanted that thing really badly. The failures? Maybe I didn't want those things as much as I thought.

If you envision a thinner version of yourself but continue to eat and drink your usual crap and only spend time thinking and dreaming, it's never going to happen. To lose the weight, you should be doing something on a daily basis to turn the dream into a reality. Dreams need to be turned into goals to come true. For example, if your dream is a holiday in Paris, it won't happen outside of your mind. But if your goal is to put $100 aside each week to go to Paris next year, bonjour gay Paree! It's the same with your physical health: Set daily or weekly goals to make the dream come true.

Past failures do not help — especially if you've lost weight in the past and looked and felt great, only to gain it again and be back where you started (fat).

The reason past experiences depress you is because you wanted to lose the weight, it was really tough, and you sacrificed many things. You pushed yourself physically to the limit and lost weight. Then, when the weight went back on, you were crushed, and now you can't stand the thought of going through all that pain again.

Look back at some of the words in that last paragraph:

- Depress
- Really tough
- Sacrificed
- Pushed to the limit
- Crushed
- Pain

My goodness, it sounds like that part of your life was a train wreck — who would want to go through that again? So don't!

"Depress"

Don't get down about it. You need to be mentally strong to be successful and if you feel sad about past failures all the time, it's never going to work.

You're overweight right now, and probably slowly putting on weight. How about making small changes to stop putting on weight? You know you need to start, so take a small, easy step right now — something that doesn't overhaul your life or get you down if it goes belly up. Stick with little changes every day, and one day the big change will come.

"Really tough"

Losing weight and getting healthy is a long-term life goal. If something is really tough, the likelihood of you getting through to the end is not as high as if it was a slight challenge. But it is achievable — just take the tough stuff out. If giving up chocolate is unbearable for you, cut back your chocolate intake. Not tough — just a slight change.

"Sacrificed"

You are not joining a convent or the priesthood here! Stop sacrificing; you won't become a martyr, so why bother? If your past diets have made you sacrifice things like going out with friends or not being able to eat your favourite foods, that is wrong and could never be a long-term solution for you.

You should be able to do everything you normally do in life and still lose weight. How? Don't sacrifice anything that is important to you — just change it. Look at what you do right now, and make an adaption: Cut back on it, replace it, and/or burn it off.

I like chocolate, and I don't mind running. I could not eat one without doing the other, or I'd put on weight, so I do both. It's not a sacrifice at all. I'm sure you could find two things in your life that go together like that. Easy!

"Pushed to the limit"

This one makes me shudder, and I've run ultra-marathons! I guess you could say I pushed myself to the limit on the days I ran them, but that was my choice, and the feeling I experienced after I finished was fantastic. But I don't run ultra-marathons daily, weekly, or even monthly. Setting yourself a long-term challenge on an activity you already like is great, but to get there, you need to train and improve. This takes you back to your little daily or weekly goals.

> 30% of Aussie cats are overweight or obese, and 40% of our pooches are too fat as well.

If you're pushing yourself to the limit every day with exercise; are drained and exhausted all the time; or if you hate what you're doing, STOP! Start off slowly, with something you can fit into your day and that makes you feel like you're working but not dying.

A 45 to 60-minute brisk walk should not push you to your limits. Once that has become a habit, give yourself another little push: Walk faster or longer, or jog a bit. When your body has accepted this, push again: Add in a gym session, a long bush walk, hills, or stairs once a week.

Each time you add something in, let your body adjust for a few weeks and then push again with something new, harder, or faster. Your PDB (Poor Dumb Body) is the best adapter: It will do anything you ask it, but it doesn't like to be beaten over the head with something new and intense. It adapts better to little changes and, in turn, it's far less painful for you.

You're probably thinking, *That's too slow; those changes will take forever to get 10 kg off.* So what? Everything you do on the movement side is burning energy, and it all adds up daily, weekly, monthly, and annually; it has to make changes to your weight, body shape, and mind, so give it the time it deserves.

"Crushed"

Feeling crushed is an awful one. You watch what you eat, you're moving more, and then — horror of horrors — you get on the scales and haven't lost any weight or, God forbid, you've put some on. You'll always feel crushed and defeated if you've struggled hard and pushed to the limits and nothing changes.

If you give yourself a year to lose some weight or turn your health and fitness around, what does one little drama on the scale mean? It doesn't mean you've had a bad week, or you're a failure — it just means the scale didn't move for you that week, or it moved slightly in the wrong direction.

Big tip: Get rid of the scale, as it's crushing you mentally. A kilo or two up and down on the scale could reflect a number of things: How much fluid you've had in the 24 hours before you got on, the time of day you weighed yourself, the amount in your bladder and bowels, the time of the month (for females), the type of scale. All these things fluctuate, but it doesn't always mean blubber and fat.

If you have to weigh yourself, do it once a month at a regular day and time and on the same scale. If you haven't lost weight in that month, at least you reversed the trend and haven't put any on — that's a thumbs-up.

If you're unhappy with the figure or put on a bit of weight, it's not the end of the world — you need to tweak your food intake and energy output on your Lazy Loser scales again. You shouldn't feel crushed if you ate better and moved a bit more. You haven't scarified anything; you just lived a better, healthier life. Keep going — you have your whole life to get it right.

"Pain"

I hate pain, and avoid it at all costs (I'm a big sook!). You should not have any hunger or other physical pains. Sure, you may feel tight and tense in the body parts you've moved more — that is normal, and will disappear as you get more used to the exercise. The best way to be pain-free is to start an activity and accept that you may have tight and sore muscles afterwards. That discomfort will go away, and when you can get through your whole session and still get out of bed in the morning, it's a sign to push yourself more and keep repeating the process. This is how your body gets fitter and stronger.

Mental-exercise rules

I've set many Lazy Loser rules in Chapter 8: Rules, and they help in a practical way if you stick to them. The same can be done with mental rules.

If you've decided you want to make a change to your eating and fitness, that's great, but it won't just happen because you put it out there to the universe. The universe has enough on its plate, and really couldn't care less about your new health regime. Make it more than a thought or a topic of conversation with your partner

On average, we're inactive 85% of the day and active 15% of it.

or a friend. Formulate a plan, stick to it until it becomes a habit, and then you're set.

• If you need to get up in the morning to exercise, set the alarm, and get up and do it.

• Write down your weekly plan in your diary and stick to it.

• Print out your weekly exercise routine, stick it on the fridge, and cross each workout off as you do it. If one isn't crossed off, that doesn't mean you skip it — give yourself 24 hours to play catch-up, then cross it off.

A few more ideas are outlined below:

Set yourself an exercise challenge.

It's easier to stay motivated when you have something to work toward. Fun runs, cycling events, and triathlons are everywhere. Many people hear those three and stick their heads under their pillows, thinking these are events for top, motivated athletes.

I've worked in the sport-and-fitness industry enough to assure you that these events are for all. In fact, there are thousands more fun runners than serious runners in any running event. These events rely on the average person who is having a go, as that is where the bulk of their entries and profits come from. They cater to all entrant levels, ages, and abilities.

Event organisers, like me, encourage all participants to train for the event they enter. Training for a fun run, cycling event, swimming event, or mini triathlon can take three to six months; in that time, you're going to get fitter and leaner. It's the training that keeps my weight on track — not race day. I tend to celebrate a little too much after my races, so the energy lost in the race is quickly replaced with high-sugar food and drink (yes, I'm talking about champagne). I still train for every event I enter, with most of my training programs lasting months. This is the part that keeps me the fittest.

Eat with your other hand! Studies show right-handed people who use their left hand to eat less!

Make sure the exercise you're doing is something you like to do.

This is important, which is why I'm always banging on about it. You're not going to do anything you don't like for very long: Just as you won't stay at a job you don't like for long or live with someone you don't like forever, you won't do an exercise or activity you don't like long term. You don't have to love it, but it needs to be something you can do and don't mind doing.

It may take a while to find what you like, so you have to trial lots of new things. That's good, because while you're trialling, you'll be using energy and getting fitter. When you start something new, stick with it for a while, as most new activities can be a bit of a challenge and you need to learn some skills first. Give it at least a month, and if it's still too hard and you aren't feeling the love (or even like), ditch it and try something new.

Rope in a buddy.

This doesn't have to be a best friend or family member. It's best if it's someone just like you: A person who wants to lose a bit of weight and get fitter, and would like some moral support. Meet three or four times a week and walk, run, or follow a Lazy Gym (see Chapter 15: Lazy Gym) program together.

It's best if this person has the same goals as you. If you rope in your partner or kids and it's not on their goal list, they may join you for a while but not be as dedicated as someone who really wants to change their health and fitness. There will be someone just like you who'd like to join in, so spread the word at your workplace, put it on your Facebook or Twitter page, etc. Someone you know will jump at the offer. Knowing you have someone waiting for you to go for a walk, run, cycle, or swim is one of the biggest motivators for exercise. Letting yourself down is a piece of cake, but letting someone else down is not as easy.

Only two other people in this world need to know your exact weight: Your doctor and the lifeboat captain.

More mental tips

You are not an animal (well, technically you are)!

But what sets us apart from other animals is the ability to use self-control. We have the power to decide yes, no, or not right now. When we want to go to the toilet, we hold on until we find a suitable place to pee (unlike our dogs that go at every tree). Every time someone annoys us, we don't slap them (well, hopefully you don't!): We practise self-control. We may feel like quitting our jobs at least once a month, but we control those feelings and work through them. However, when it comes to resisting the temptation to eat, we say we have no self-control!

What you need to understand is that by not resisting that extra serving of dessert, you face consequences: You get fatter, unhealthier, and unhappier. Surely those consequences are just as harmful as the other ones from what we do control in our lives.

Self-control is not a new concept to you. You probably apply self-control every hour of your life — so do it with food and drink.

When we use self-control, it usually involves a bit of internal dialogue:

"I need a pee."

Internal talk: *I think I can get through this meeting without wetting myself, so I'll wait. Or, Not sure where the nearest toilet is...oh well, I'll hold on until I get home.*

"I can't stand this guy . . . I could just slap him."

Internal talk: *Here he goes, going on and on. Oh well . . . it'll be over soon, and he'll be out of my face. Just smile and look fascinated.*

"Work's driving me crazy! I'm thinking of telling them where to stick it today."

Internal talk: *Well, it's been really busy; when things settle down it will be better again. Or, I go on holiday in a few weeks, so that is something to look forward to. Or, The money's good — how would I pay the mortgage if I quit?*

Yet where food and drink is concerned, we turn into the Cookie Monster: It's there; I have to have it now. Coooookieeeee!

Try internal talk when you're faced with food temptations:

"Yay, it's morning tea time!"

Internal talk: *Do I need something to eat or drink now, or can I wait until lunchtime? Or, Do I need a flat white now, or am I just thirsty? Maybe a glass of water is enough. Or, I could do with something, but I'm sure it could be half a snack to get me to lunchtime.*

"I gotta have that last piece of chocolate cake!"

Internal talk: *Why not wait until the kids get home and share it with them? I still get a taste, but I'm not scoffing the whole lot — and I'm sure that will make them happy.*

"I need a drink."

Internal talk: *I've had a shocking day and I could do with something, but if I open that wine, I'm not sure I could stop at just one. Why not bypass the drink cabinet, put on my sports gear, ring up Jo, and go for a good walk and talk to get it all out of my system?*

Every time you feel like eating and drinking, think for a bit. If you have your internal dialogue and still think, *What the hell — I want it and I'm having it,* then go for it. But the longer you think before you scoff, the more self-control you'll apply on other occasions. Just like I discuss in Chapter 3: Fat Habits, self-control is a habit — the more you apply it, the better you get at it, and after a while it becomes second nature.

Why were women in the 1950s thinner than today's ladies without going to the gym and exercising? They didn't need to: They burned an average of 1,000 calories a day on domestic duties, while today's women use half that amount of energy on housework. The 1950s woman did three hours of housework a day, took a two-hour round-trip walk to shops, and spent an hour preparing dinner and cleaning up afterward. Most of them didn't have access to the family car, so they also walked children to and from school. Plus, they ate fewer calories — the average daily calorie consumption was 1,818 in the 1950s for a woman; today, it's about 2,178 calories.

And also, like I say in Chapter 8: Rules, even if you only use self-control on half the occasions when you have yummy food choices, that's still better than gobbling everything in your line of sight all the time.

Be nicer to Number One: You!

How many times do you tell yourself how great you are in a day?

And how many times do your berate or criticise yourself in that same day?

Add it up, and then, like your Lazy Loser scales, invent some Lazy Mental ones: Negative thoughts about yourself go in the left-hand side, and positive ones go in the right-hand side. Is the left side denting the bench and the right swinging in the breeze? That is often the case with people who are unhappy with their lives or bodies.

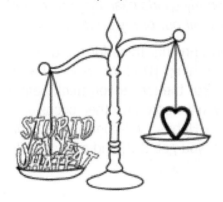

You can apply your Lazy Loser rules here, too. During the day, take out a thought from the left-hand side and turn it into something that can fit into the right hand side. For example:

Left side: *I'm fat and hopeless.*

Right side: *No one is hopeless, so I can't be that. I'm overweight, though, and I'm working on changing that on a daily basis.*

Left side: *I just ate that last Tim Tam. I'm such a disgrace.*

Right side: *Stealing from the blind beggar on the street is a disgrace; eating a Tim Tam is normal. I've done it, so now I have to find a way to get rid of it — today. Looks like a long walk is coming after dinner.*

Left side: *I'm never going to drop 10 kg by my 20-year school reunion in five weeks. I'm such an idiot.*

Right side: *I'm not an idiot, which is how I know quite well that I can't lose 10 kg in five weeks. What about 10 kg in 12 months?*

Criticism is being mean to yourself — don't do that. So you ate the last chocolate biscuit on the plate. Are you going to tell yourself off all day? Because nasty words don't make you burn calories. However, a brisk, angry walk or boxing session will do it.

We're good at dishing out praise to others; even if we don't think that person has done something amazing, we tend to over-exaggerate our praise of them. Yet when it comes to ourselves, we go the other way: We underestimate our worth all the time. What happens when we're sad and miserable and have been telling ourselves off all day? On the way home: "Oh look, there's my favourite takeaway joint. I'm going through the drive-thru, because I need some cheering up." But what comes after the yummy, greasy takeaway? More criticism and self-loathing. It's a vicious cycle, with you getting fatter each time around.

I've found one great way to solve this: Talk about yourself in the third person. Pretend you are your best mate, or one of your kids, or your poor old mum. I do it all the time now, and it really works.

Psychologists say that when we start using the "I" word, many statements become negative: "I'm hopeless", "I'm an idiot", "I stuffed up", etc. The way to turn it around is to pretend you're talking about someone else, like a friend.

For instance, say you've lost a bit of weight, but your goal was to lose double that in the timeframe you set for yourself. You've had a couple of blowouts, but most of the time you've been really focused on eating well and exercising more.

The "I" in you would say, "I'm so disappointed in myself. I've lost a bit of weight, but I should've lost more. I had a binge session on junk food last weekend, and that really got me down. Sometimes I think it's hardly worth it."

Now, your best friend comes to you with the same sad story as yours. Would this be your response?

Any food bought from a charity — pie drives, chocolate drives, girls' guide cookies, etc. — and anything eaten at a neighbourhood watch meeting should contain zero calories.

"Yes, I agree, you're hopeless. I don't know why you even bother."
You know you would never say that to someone else, and are more
likely to say this:

"Hey, come on, don't be so hard on yourself. You've lost weight,
and that's what it's all about. So you had a pig-out — we all do
— but look how well you got back on track, and you're looking
fantastic. I can really tell that you've lost weight."

Remember, this is an internal conversation, so no one is going to
overhear and say, "Wow, who's got a few tickets on themselves,
then?"

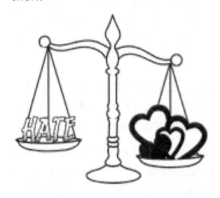

Positive words create nice
feelings. You don't have to
believe them, or you can think
they are exaggerated, but that
doesn't matter — when we hear
a compliment about ourselves,
we get warm, fuzzy feelings. And
it also doesn't matter who makes
the compliment — a stranger,
the 16-year-old serving you in the
clothes shop, your best friend, partner, boss, or even yourself. No
matter where it comes from, it feels good. Make yourself your best
mate, and start talking to yourself like a buddy would.

Stop making food Number One

Food is not a real being — you do know that, don't you?

It's not your best friend, buddy, or lover. You're not married to it,
and it isn't your arch nemesis; food doesn't care two hoots about
you. It tastes good and sometimes makes us feel good, but there
are lots of other things in our lives that are so much better than
food: People, jobs, pets, and babies are some of the things that
are wonderful, and yet all we focus on all day is the big chocolate
cake we plan to binge on tonight.

One thing I've noticed while working in the health-and-fitness
industry is the way many people continually think and obsess
about food. Food is just stuff we eat to keep us moving, and yet it

possesses some people's thoughts every waking hour. How did it get to the top of the tree in our lives?

Test yourself: What do you think about when you wake up in the morning? Is it what you're going to eat or not eat all day, or something else? If it's the former, you need to stop doing that.

When I wake up, my thoughts are one of two things. If I'm going for a run, then I get up and go. If I'm not running, I wake up with thoughts of what I have to do that day, whether I'll fit it all in and, if so, in what order? Yes, I think of food — but only when I'm hungry and want my breakfast.

Obsessing and thinking about food and what you're going to eat constantly is a bad habit like all the ones in Chapter 3: Fat Habits. How do you stop? Like with all habits, you replace it with another one.

Find a new hobby or obsession. Somewhere down the road, you were probably on a new diet, which is like a new hobby. At the start, it's exciting, as you have lots of new things to think about and are busy planning out your future super-skinny life. You spend the day thinking about food plans, serving sizes, and calorie counting, and it's wonderful. However, it probably crashed and burned like all diets, but the food obsession stuck with you and became your new hobby: When and where and what your next food hit is going to be.

Now it's time to get over that hobby and find a new one.

You probably know I'm going to suggest a hobby like exercise (yes, you know me too well). This is because it's a double whammy: You stop obsessing about food, and you move more. For example:

Old hobby: You usually watch the clock at work all morning for lunchtime, so you can race down to the local café and order your latte and toasted ham-and-cheese focaccia.

The following are the most common reasons people break their diets: A divorce or breakup, getting married, getting fired, being promoted, being at your mother's house, eating out, eating in, your birthday, someone else's birthday, you've stuck to your diet for four weeks, Valentine's day, holidays, and the list goes on and on.

New hobby: You're going to go swimming on your lunch break. Your new morning thoughts are: *Have I got all my gear with me? How many laps will I fit in on my lunch break? And, If I go a bit faster, I might be able to squeeze another couple in.*

Old hobby: From 3 p.m. on, all you can think about is Drink O'Clock at 6 p.m. — and maybe a few nibbles to go with it.

New hobby: Go home quickly and get changed, as you're starting your new Pilates class at 6 p.m.

Your new hobby doesn't have to be exercise; there's probably something you've always wanted to do or learn but never got around to. Learn a musical instrument, take a writing course, adopt a new puppy from the dog shelter — pick anything you like, and slot it in for the time of the day you obsess about or crave food. If you wake up to your new puppy crying because he needs to go out for a walk, all thoughts of food disappear.

When you think about food over the day, stop and deliberately change your thoughts to something else or distract yourself and do something else. This can be hard, but you have to work on it. For instance, if you think about food, get up and walk outside and come back in; read one page of your book; ring a friend and have a chat; or clean something. If you keep this up, soon the food thoughts will be replaced with other things.

Emotional eating

If you've picked up my vibe throughout this book, you probably think I'd fling this one in with those nonsense excuses people use when it comes to defending their bad eating and exercise habits. So it may shock you when I say that emotional eating is a real thing — it happens, and is very hard to break. It is not an excuse, but it is a big fat habit — and as you found out in Chapter 3: Fat Habits, all habits are breakable.

Somewhere along your life track (it could even have been when you were a toddler), food was used to make you feel better. You fell over and scraped a knee, and you were given a lollipop for being such a brave boy or girl. As a teenager, you may have had a bad day at school, so you came home and comforted yourself with lots of yummy food. Your parents may have rewarded good work with taking you out for a meal or buying you food treats. All these things made you turn to food when you felt down, bad, or hurt.

Then there are people who eat more when they're happy. They haven't a care in the world, and they go out and indulge more. They feel good about themselves, so they treat themselves with food rewards. They're happiest when they're with their family and friends, and often these occasions are built around getting together for meals and drinks. Every situation is a source of celebration, so eat, drink, and be merry.

Is one of these you? Do you eat more when you're down, or go out more when you're happy, which leads to eating and drinking more?

I can't make you feel better about yourself, but what I can tell you is that you got into a habit with your emotional eating. When you're sad, eating may make you feel better in the moment — when the chocolate is melting in your mouth and sliding down your throat. After that, you feel not so happy. Then what? You eat more to feel happier.

If you're eating emotionally on a daily basis because you're sad every day, get some help. You shouldn't be sad every day. Go to your doctor and tell him or her that you feel sad more than you feel happy. Your doctor will set you on the right path to get help.

If your emotions fluctuate over the month and you eat lots of comfort food during the low moments, you can change that. Use the tricks above on obsessing about food. When you feel sad or flat, don't eat — move. Leave the house or your workplace and walk away, and then of course walk back when the feeling has passed.

If you eat more when you're stressed, replace the food with exercise. Pushing yourself to a hot sweat is the best thing for stress; I do it all the time. I imagine the sweat is all the stress seeping out of my body, and it really works.

The only person you're ever required to stand naked in front of is a prison guard (an excellent reason to try to stay out of jail).

If you're a happy eater, that's okay. But if you're happy and eating 24/7, that's a bad habit. Look at the food you're eating: If it's high in sugar, it could be the sweet hit giving you a happy rush and causing you to crave more food. Change your happy eating to healthy eating, and you may find the old way of eating was more about the sweets than your feeling of constant delight.

If you crave food when you're happy, sad, or stressed, eat a carrot. Try this for a while; every time you want to eat because of an emotion, reach for a carrot or celery stick. I'm not telling you to do this because they are healthy, low-calorie options; after a while of turning to plain old veggies when you feel an emotion, you'll soon see there's really no comfort in food. It will bore you, and you'll associate those feelings with food that's not so exciting or even comforting.

Guilt

"I feel so guilty, but what the hell — one more won't hurt." I hear this often when people are offered yummy food. I'm not sure if they say it because they feel overweight and think the person offering the food may be judging them for eating a treat, or because they really do feel guilty.

You may feel guilty for forgetting someone's birthday, yelling at the kids, or murdering someone, but beating yourself up over eating food is crazy. Other guilt can be sorted: You can send a belated birthday card, apologise to the kids, or spend the rest of your life in jail, but how do you assuage food guilt?

Guilt is another negative emotion that makes you feel bad, and will never help you on your quest for a happy, healthy life. To put such a strong emotion on food is silly; remember: Food is a nobody, so stop giving it such a high-ranking role in your life.

Once you've eaten something you feel you shouldn't have, don't turn it into a drama. Done is done, so think forward: The extra bit you gobbled will leave your system sooner or later, and if you don't want it to leave tell-tale signs that it was ever there — meaning you want to get rid of the guilty evidence — then move it or make a deal with it.

You ate the last chocolate biscuit? Get out and walk, run, or work in the garden for half an hour. You gorged on a family pizza last night? No fast food for the rest of the week. You got stuck into the grog on the weekend? Looks like you're riding the bike to work next week — no car.

I guess you could say this is your jail sentence; however, it's better than beating yourself up and getting down about something you ate and can't take back.

Remember your Lazy Loser scales: When you have a splurge you have put something into the left-hand side. Once it's in there, it can't come off — the only solution is to add something to the right-hand side, and it needs to be done within 24 hours to get the balance back again. No guilt — just payback.

Lazy Bottom Line

• We eat for lots of reasons, and it seems that hunger is not at the top of the list anymore. If you're eating for reasons other than starvation prevention, find out why and what your food weakness is. Make small changes to stop it from making you put on weight.

• If you're jaded from past weight-loss experiences, put it all in the past: Start fresh and move on.

• Stop putting too much thought and emphasis on food and drink in your life. Take it down a few levels — make it less than a four on your top-10 priority list, and keep moving it down to a low-priority thought.

• Emotional eating is habit. If you turn to food when you're sad, happy, or stressed, you need to replace it with something else that will help you deal with those feelings. However, if you eat more on a daily basis because you're sad most of the time, talk to someone who can help you with your sadness.

If someone asks you, "When are you due?" and you're not pregnant, just reply, "Any minute now!"

• Don't start or continue on an eating or exercise plan that makes you feel deprived, depressed, or in pain; it will never work in the long term.

• Try not to berate yourself constantly about the food you eat or the weight you are right now. Criticism doesn't help anyone, and will not work for you. Practice saying more nice than nasty things in a day. Tally it up at the end of each day, so you can keep track and make thought changes.

• Replace thoughts of food with other thoughts or actions. Get a new hobby — be like Elvis and leave the building (well, maybe Elvis is a bad example, as he obviously didn't leave his building enough!). Read, chat, sing — anything to change food thoughts.

• Stop being Cookie Monster with food and apply the self-control you use in other areas of your life. Never reach for something without having a little chat with yourself first. If you have the internal debate and still decide you're going for it, then do — but at least you can say you put thought into it before you gobbled.

If you ask a man, "Does my butt look big in this?", never expect an answer you can live with.

Chapter 17 – What Type of Loser Are You?

I started Lazy Loser four years ago, and I've had lots of Losers in that time (that's a good thing!). And although my clients have had different issues with their weight and fitness, I've noticed some commonalities among them.

Regardless of sex, age, size, lifestyle, and culture, most of the Losers' eating patterns fell into five categories. I gathered which type each Loser was from the food and exercise diaries they filled in during their first week, and pigeonholed them from that. There were a few square pegs, and some Losers could easily have fit into more than one group; however, in the majority of cases, a dominant eating characteristic led them to their Loser groups.

Classifying the Loser type made it easy for me to be able to offer some tips and advice on their little peccadillos rather than just clump them all into the one "Let's lose weight now!" category.

Knowing why you're fat and what your weaknesses are and how to tweak them is the start of becoming the Lazy Loser you want to be.

I've said many times throughout this book that weight gain is due to eating too much and not expending enough energy. Finding out the way we eat too much, what we eat too much of, and how we eat can affect the way we start changing our eating patterns.

Lazy Loser categories:

1. Tipsy Loser

2. Moo Loser

3. Sweet Loser

4. Super Loser

5. Piggy Loser

I wonder if you can guess which each means from their labels. If you're like me, you may be thinking, Yes, *all of the above, thank you,* but I bet you're likelier to fall into one category more than the others.

The following pages will enlighten you. Read about each category, and when you recognise yourself, not only will you see what type of Loser you are, but you'll also find out how to work on your eating foibles and, hopefully without too much angst, change a few of them.

All the examples and eating plans are from real-life Lazy Losers I've worked with over the past few years. I will not reveal their names — not because of confidentiality or privacy, but because I think my names are a lot funnier than theirs!

Tipsy Loser

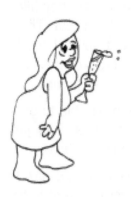

Being a Tipsy Loser doesn't make you an alcoholic, but for the purpose of this section, if you like a drink and you can't lose weight, you're a Tipsy Loser!

I want to reiterate: No food or drink is bad. You won't see me bashing you over the head with your empty wine bottle, telling you how naughty you are. However, alcohol, like many things we consume, can have health risks. It's always a good idea to keep a close eye on your alcohol consumption, but yes, you can drink while on a Lazy Loser program.

Tell-tale signs of a Tipsy Loser?

• You have a wine or beer with dinner at least three times a week

• You don't drink during the week but you go out on weekends and get wasted!

• You drink at least 4 standard alcoholic drinks a week

• You can't remember the last time a week went by in which you didn't drink

• Most days you have your alarm set for drink (or wine or beer) O'clock

• You can never resist a Happy Hour

Sample day plan of a Tipsy Loser

Breakfast: She's too busy to eat, so Tipsy grabs coffee on the run and makes up for it at morning tea.

Morning tea: Muffin and coffee

Lunch: Salad sandwich and coffee

Afternoon tea: Nil

Pre-dinner: G and T with nibbles

Dinner: Grilled chicken, two small potatoes, steamed veggies

Drink: Two glasses of white wine

Dessert: Two scoops of ice cream with chocolate topping

I told Tipsy Loser to list everything she had to eat and drink, along with the quantities. However, as you can see, it's quite vague — maybe she had too much to drink the night before! Therefore, I get Tipsy to clarify a few things:

• It was a big chocolate muffin for morning tea.

• The salad sandwich was bought from the café near work (Tipsy Loser buys lunch here every day). It was premade and had ham, salad, butter, a slice of cheese, and mayonnaise on wholemeal bread.

Only 1% of the population can get away with wearing a thong; chances are you are not in this percentage bracket.

- Nibbles were pistachios shared with a partner. She's not sure how many they ate, but her partner ate far more.

- Tipsy Loser thinks it was a shot of gin; when told a shot is 30 ml, Tipsy Loser thought it could have been one and a half shots.

- It was two large glasses of wine.

Tipsy Loser left off energy output, and said she did nothing that day. Nothing?

I asked Tipsy Loser if that was due to a hangover, and she laughed. Then, with a bit more thought, she remembered that she rode her bike to work (which is one of the reasons she missed breakfast): 45 minutes to work and 45 minutes back home. Tipsy Loser's job is half sedentary and half active: The active bit sees her running around town like a "Chook with its head cut off" (Tipsy's description, not mine).

Many of the Lazy Loser plans I get back can be vague, reasons for this fall under these four categories:

A. I forgot what I ate and drank.

B. I don't want to remember what I ate and drank.

C. I'm in denial about what I ate and drank.

D. I'm embarrassed to reveal what I ate and drank.

On the energy side, we often forget the incidental exercise, or think it's not important enough to mention.

Tipsy's tweaks

Breakfast: You must have brekkie, even if it's a piece of fruit. Cereal or yoghurt, are good — they're quick, and require no cooking.

Morning tea: No baked products. Take something with you from home (e.g. fruit, yoghurt, nuts).

A naked body looks 2 kg slimmer in the dark. Subtract another 2 kg if you're on your back and an extra 5 kg if you're under the covers.

Lunch: Stick with the café, but don't get a premade roll or wrap — get one freshly made.

Here are the rules with salad rolls, sandwiches, or wraps: Choose butter/margarine or mayonnaise — not both —one spread is plenty. Two spreads counteract each other, and you won't taste one above the other. This is a cheap calorie saver.

Have meat or cheese, not both. Same as above: You can usually only taste one or the other, and won't notice one is missing. You may like to alternate on different days: Meat and salad one day, cheese and salad the next.

Pre-dinner: One shot of gin after work (and if you don't mind your mixers, go for the low-calorie or sugar-free ones), and count out nibbles: 20 — pistachios, macadamias, Brazil nuts, small rice snacks, or chips. No, that's not 100 nibbles — you have to pick one type. Make sure all snacks are unsalted; salted foods make you thirsty and want to drink more.

Now the elephant: Alcohol. Tipsy Loser revealed she'd been having a G and T and a couple of glasses of wine every night for years. She does have alcohol-free days every now and again, but not weekly. She loves a drink — it keeps Tipsy Loser sane.

There are two choices for Tipsy Loser (drinkers should always have choices!):

1. Keep the G and T (gin and tonic), but make sure there's only one shot (30 ml) of gin or less in it. Put half a chopped-up lemon or lime in the glass, and you won't miss the half shot.

2. If you must have a drink with dinner every night, have one glass of wine only. If you want to have two glasses a night, then you need to have wine with dinner every other night. There — you've just halved your wine intake.

New Tipsy Loser eating plan

Breakfast: Piece of fruit and small tub of low-fat yoghurt.

Morning tea: 20 unsalted large nuts.

Lunch: Salad sandwich or roll (wholemeal), made to order: Meat, tuna, or chicken and salad, with no cheese and a choice of butter or mayo (not both).

Afternoon tea: Piece of fruit.

Pre-dinner: G and T (one shot with a low-calorie mixer, lots of ice, and lemon) with 20 large unsalted nuts. Pistachios are good, as Tipsy has to work to eat them, and that slows her down a bit!

Dinner: Red meat, chicken, or fish with veggies — all good here. This meal is the best of the day, so I didn't want to tamper with the one that was healthy and filling.

Drink: A choice between two glasses of wine tonight and none tomorrow night, or one glass tonight and one tomorrow night.

Dessert: One scoop of ice cream with chocolate topping.

Results on Tipsy's Lazy Loser scales

Left side: Food and drink

• Added in breakfast, but took out a large chunk of morning-tea calories.

• Took two things off the salad roll.

• Cut grazing dramatically (I'd say by half).

• Cut alcohol in half.

That's a lot off the input side!

Right side: Output

Tipsy rides to and from work each day (approximately 90 minutes a day of easy riding). She doesn't do any other exercise during the week, as she hasn't got time. However, on the weekend, Tipsy Loser will walk for an hour each day.

I didn't change the output too much; Tipsy Loser works nine-hour days, life is hectic from Monday to Friday, and she does ride her bike twice a day. Walking on the weekend means she is adding something onto the output side. I suggested she increase her weekend walks by 15 minutes and walk faster.

> Never allow anyone to take your photo while you're eating, drinking, squatting, bending over, playing limbo or twister, dancing, or jumping into a pool.

Feedback after one week of changes

"I survived — and it was easy, as I was not off the alcohol long enough to miss it. I went with two glasses of wine every other day, as I felt it would be good to have some alcohol-free days; I didn't even have the G and T on those days. Having breakfast made a big difference to the morning-tea pig-out. And yes, 20 nuts was enough for pre-dinner nibbles."

Most importantly, Tipsy Loser didn't feel deprived or hungry, and could see herself doing this forever; in her mind, it was a bit of tweaking.

Tips for Tipsy Losers

1. Measure out shots of alcohol: One shot is 30 ml. Trial 15 ml shots — you probably won't notice the difference.

2. Add lots of ice and fruit (lemons or limes) to your mixed-drink glass before you put the alcohol in.

3. Use zero-calorie or soda-water mixers.

4. Alternate alcohol and water (i.e., one glass of wine, beer, or cider and one glass of water, then a glass of alcohol again). Drink the water as slowly as you drank your glass of alcohol.

5. Use wine glasses or champagne flutes when you drink water: It will feel like you're having a real drink.

6. If you're a beer drinker, try shandies with soda water (half beer, half soda); the same can be done with alcoholic ciders.

7. If you're a champagne drinker, put three strawberries in the flute first and then pour the champagne, which will cut the alcohol in half.

8. Drink your alcohol slowly. Look at the clock, and make each drink last for at least half an hour.

9. We relax more when we drink, which means our self-control can go out the window and we tend to eat more. Make it a rule not to eat while drinking. Have your drink before or after your meal. If you can't resist a snack with your drink you can have 10 nuts or 10 chips per glass of alcohol — no more.

10. Don't drink at home, or opt to have no alcohol in your house (and no, that doesn't mean you eat out every night). Set a rule that you only drink when you go to a restaurant, hotel, or when you're invited to a friend's house, so maybe only once or twice a week. This is good way to cut back on alcohol consumption.

11. Don't drink alone (another good rule if you find yourself doing this often).

Moo Loser

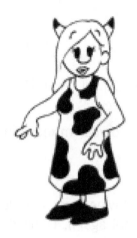

I have you guessing now: *What can a Moo Loser be? Am I one?*

I grew up on a dairy farm, and remember lying in long grassy fields and watching our cows. I'd given them all names! I marvelled at how slow and content they seemed to be, but mostly I loved the way they ate. They ate all day. They even ate when they were being milked twice a day. No breakfast, lunch, and dinner here: It was an all-day graze.

You guessed it: Moo Loser is a grazer. During most of the daylight hours and some of the dark hours, Moo Loser is chewing on something.

Moo Losers are tricky, as they do not eat out of hunger. They eat from habit, boredom, comfort, you name it — just graze, graze, graze.

It's tough to pin Moos down for a Lazy Loser plan, as they nibble so much throughout the day they can't possibly remember it all. But of course the calories are not forgotten. The upside to Moos is that unlike my farm friends, they tend to be a bit more active. Up down, in and out, getting food, preparing food, eating food — all high-energy stuff.

Tell-tale signs of a Moo Loser?

• You put something in your mouth at least every hour of your waking day

• You often eat left overs

• You eat at your desk or in front of a computer or TV daily

• You love snacks

• You taste food off other peoples plates

• You eat in the car daily

• You often eat whilst standing up or walking

• At the end of the day you have forgotten all the amount of snacks you have eaten

• You lick spoons, knives and your fingers at least once a day

Sample day plan of a Moo Loser

Breakfast: Two poached eggs on toast, along with the crusts off someone else's toast before it gets thrown out.

Between breakfast and morning tea:

• While preparing lunches: A snippet of ham, an extra slice of cheese accidentally cut with no room on the sandwich, and a lick of the mayo knife.

• A few Tic-Tacs on the drive to work (found in the car).

• Black coffee and a few broken biscuits from the bottom of the cookie jar as soon as she's in the office.

• Someone gave a fruit basket to the business, so a bunch of grapes to nibble on.

100 g of dried bananas have 2210 kj — that is equal to nine bananas!

Morning tea: Two more biscuits, with coffee.

Lunch: Soup and wholemeal roll with coffee.

Afternoon tea: More of the fruit basket (a bit of this and that, all healthy). Offered half a muffin by another staff member.

Kids' swimming lessons after work: Little Moo insisted she wanted a bag of Twisties. She ran off to play with a buddy, then got back and howled because they were all gone! Moo stopped at the supermarket quickly to get dinner items, and a lovely staff member offered dry biscuits with a new dip. Moo ate three samples.

Pre-dinner: She cooked roast lamb with all the trimmings, had a couple of slices of meat to see if it was cooked properly, had to keep testing gravy, and had a roast potato to check if it was cooked perfectly as well.

Dinner: Moo only had a small serving, as she wasn't feeling so hungry.

After dinner: The Little Moos never eat all their veggies, so she polished those off before putting plates in the dishwasher. She finally gets to sit down and have a rest.

Dessert: Reward for a busy day? A hot chocolate and two marshmallows. With the marshmallow bag opened, she had a few more, but didn't count how many.

As for energy out, Moo Loser is always busy. Although she has an office job, she's up and down all day (I wonder why) and spends most out-of-work hours running after kids. Moo is also a runner and is training for a marathon, so she runs four days a week, totalling 50 km or more.

Moo's tweaks

Eating all the time isn't good for you. Once you've satisfied your body of its need for food, you should let it do what it's supposed to do. Digest the food and send the nutrients and energy to the working muscles, organs, and systems in the body; if it's digesting food all day, it's working overtime.

Be in control of what and how much you eat. Allocate all snacks and nibbles at the start of the day and when they're gone, snacking and nibbling is over.

Lazy Loser

Don't eat anyone else's food; leftovers on someone else's plate are not for you. Get each family member to clear their own plates when they're finished, so you won't be tempted.

New Moo Loser eating plan

Breakfast: Moo eats a healthy breakfast that should set her up for the day and keep hunger at bay, therefore I say stick to the eggs on toast. But Moo has a new rule: She's not to eat anything that wasn't prepared for her, so no kids' scraps or other people's leftovers.

Between breakfast and morning tea: Moo Loser has to take a bunch of grapes or other small pieces of cut-up fruit with her to work, and that is the only thing she can snack on between meals. Once the fruit is gone, the snacking is over, so she needs to make them last.

Morning tea: Coffee and one biscuit from the tin.

Lunch: The soup and roll is a good, healthy meal.

Afternoon tea: Again, Moo has to make the grapes or fruit pieces last.

Kids' swimming lessons after work: Moo goes prepared. She takes fruit, and tells Little Moo that's all she's having. That way, when she runs off to play, Moo can nibble on the fruit, which is healthy for both her and Little Moo. As for how to deal with tantrums (not yours, the kids') that arise at snack shops, say you have no money. I used to lie to my kids all the time — it works! Show them your empty purse and say, "Oops, sorry — I haven't got any money left for Twisties, but I have some fruit in my bag."

Dinner: Any dinner she likes that is healthy for her and the family. Running requires a good dose of carbohydrates and protein, so meat, pasta or rice, and veggies are great. She can taste test while cooking, but only with a teaspoon; it's a taste, not a snack.

Dessert: Hot chocolate made with skim milk and five marshmallows, eaten slowly: One every 10 minutes.

> We spend an average of three to four hours a day resisting things we desire (and I didn't say it was all food)!

After dessert, Moo brushes her teeth. Eating has ceased until tomorrow morning: Breakfast time.

Results on Moo's Lazy Loser scales

Left side: Food and drink

- Took out all the leftover nibbles.
- Cut grazing dramatically (I'd say by half).

That's a good dent in the input scale!

Right side: Output

Moo is following a running training program at the moment and I didn't want to jeopardise that with any new activities, so I didn't change the output. 40 to 50 km a week of running and chasing after kids the rest of the time is plenty of energy output.

Feedback after one week of changes

"The rules worked! When I told myself I wasn't going to eat any of the kids' scraps or leftover food, I found I really stuck to it. The bunch of grapes at work were a great idea — I did snack, but only on them, so at the end of the day I knew exactly what I'd eaten; usually I have no idea! And yes, lying works: No money, so no snacks at swimming. Overall it was easy, and I was really pleased with myself at the end of each day, knowing I had showed more self-control with my grazing."

Tips for Moo Losers

1. Only eat when you're sitting down. This is tough, as you have to determine whether you have time to sit and eat all day. Check when you're about to put something in your mouth: You have to be sitting.

2. Don't eat other people's leftovers. If you can't throw food in the bin, give it to the dog, make it compost, or get someone else to clear the dinner plates each night.

3. Prepare your grazing snack at the start of the day. Take a bag of grapes or a box of sultanas with you for grazing on, and nothing else. Once they're gone, your daily grazing is over.

4. Be anal about your grazing: You're only allowed to have a grazing snack every half hour, set the clock for it. After one grape, when the clock ticks over half an hour, you can have another grape; do this until you break your grazing habit.

5. Set up food-free zones at home and work. Make your desk a food-free zone, so if you want to eat, you have to leave your desk and go searching for food. At home, make the food-free zone the TV room; each time you want a snack, you have to go to the kitchen, sit there by yourself with no entertainment, and eat it.

6. Don't eat while driving. No food in the car (not even mints).

7. Brush your teeth right after dinner, so you can't eat or drink anything else for the rest of the night.

Sweet Loser

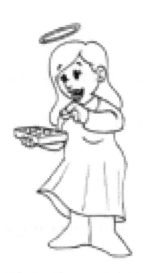

This one sounds nice (maybe yummy is a better word).

You love all things sweet, are a self-confessed chocolate addict, and have a few little stashes all over the house! You're scared to go on a diet, as you know you'll be told to ditch the chocolate . . . which means life will be miserable, and you won't survive!

Before we start, let's get this big chestnut off the table: Chocolate is not addictive, so you can stop throwing that out there as your excuse. Yes, its yummy, we love it, and it makes us feel good, but we don't have to have it. We don't need a support group for it (although I would be up for a social chocolate-eating get together every now and again if I could do so anonymously!). Alcohol, nicotine, and caffeine are addictive, but not chocolate. However, that doesn't stop it from being tantalisingly delicious!

Tell-tale signs of a Sweet Loser?

• You love chocolates, lollies, cakes, and sweet muffins

• You eat chocolate daily

• You crave sweet food

• You think chocolate is better than sex!

• You like sweet drinks as well; sugar in tea or coffee, hot chocolate, flavoured drinks or soft drinks

• You claim you are addicted to chocolate

• Dessert is your favourite meal of the day

Sample day plan of a Sweet Loser

Breakfast: Two slices of thick raisin toast with jam.

Morning tea: Two Tim Tams.

Lunch: Bowl of salad.

Afternoon tea: Two homemade chocolate-chip cookies when the kids get home from school.

Dinner: Chicken stir-fry (lots of veggies with rice).

Dessert #1: Five pieces of chocolate.

Dessert #2: Another homemade chocolate-chip cookie.

Dessert #3: Two more pieces of chocolate.

Oh dear. It started off so well, but quickly slid into the sweet gutter by morning tea.

For energy output, Sweet Loser walks the baby and kids to school in the morning and afternoon: 15 minutes each way at a slow pace. She kept busy most of day with housekeeping and childcare. The baby is six months old, and Sweet Loser hasn't gotten back

Australians eat only 6 kg of eggs per year, per person. Japan and Denmark are the best googy eaters at 19 kg, followed by Mexico at 18 kg.

into an exercise routine yet; she's going back to work in three months, and isn't sure if she should go back to her usual gym-class exercise routine.

I asked Sweet Loser for the lowdown on her eating, and she told me that once she starts eating something sweet, she can't stop. Sweet Loser also bakes lots of sweet treats for school lunches, and can't resist them when they come out of the oven — or sometimes before they even go in, like licking the bowl or eating the raw cookie dough.

Sweet Loser feels she eats healthy in all other ways except for this sweet addiction. She doesn't look for sweet drinks or other snacks — it's just baked sweet foods or good-old-fashioned chocolate. I asked her if there was a Dessert #4, and didn't get an answer.

I really felt for Sweet Loser: This was me 20 years ago. Yes, I was the wonderful mum of four kids who cooked up delightful treats for my darlings after school. If only they knew what I served up to them was only half of what came out of the oven. I'd buy family-size blocks of chocolate and hide them from the kids so I could give it out as treats, but guess what? My kids never got treats. And then I'd congratulate myself for eating all the bad stuff and keeping my babies healthy. "How come you didn't get fat?" you ask. I was running by then, and probably not eating enough at other meals, but that didn't make it a healthy diet — and I always knew that in the back of my mind.

Sweet's tweaks

I wanted to allow Sweet Loser to have some chocolate, as I thought she'd feel deprived without it. But she needed to curb the start time and the binging, and follow these rules:

• No sweets until the after-school sharing.

• Sweet Loser was having too little at lunch and leaving room and hunger for the sweet snacks she was planning to binge on— she has to eat a decent lunch.

• She needs a distraction from all the yummy stuff in the house. Take the baby for a mid-morning walk for half an hour to an hour — right at that Tim Tam moment.

- Sweet Loser needs to get back into an exercise routine; walking between 30 and 60 minutes a day after having a baby is ideal. Plus, she may be ready to slowly get back into her gym work: She should try one session a week on weekends to ease her way back into them.

- Sad to say, but Sweet Loser has to curb the culinary skills. Cookies, muffins, and chocolate slices are yummy, but there are many other yummy alternatives that the kids will love.

- Sweet Loser needs to stop making cakes, muffins, and slices out of cocoa, white flour, cooking chocolate, cream, and eggs. She can use ingredients like oats, muesli, nuts (if no allergies), wholegrain flour, and low-fat milks for baking. Then, if she likes the chocolate look, she can melt chocolate and use it as thin icing. It looks chocolaty, tastes chocolaty, but is so much better for her and the children.

New Sweet Loser eating plan

Breakfast: Two poached eggs on toast. No honey, jam, or other sweet things for breakfast, as that starts the sugar craving too early in the day.

Morning tea: Piece of fruit (e.g., apple, orange, pear, banana), then off for a walk with baby.

Lunch: Vegetable soup and a wholemeal roll.

Afternoon tea: A piece of the new, healthy baked slice with the kids after school.

Dinner: Chicken stir-fry (lots of veggies with rice); this can stay the same, as it's all good.

Dessert #1: One scoop of chocolate ice cream (low-fat, if desired).

Dessert # 2: One small piece of the new baked slice.

Desserts #3 and #4: Nil and ditto.

There are no surprises here: Aussies love their bananas. We each eat about 624 bananas annually, and our fruit consumption sits at 106 kg per person.

Results on Sweet's Lazy Loser scales

Left side: Food and drink

• Changed the sweet breakfast to savoury to stop the sweet craving from starting too early in the day.

• Took out the Tim Tams.

• Halved the chocolate treats.

• Cut back the after-dinner splurge.

That's a lot off the input scales!

Right side: Output

Sweet Loser needed a bit more of push with her energy output. It's hard to get back into it when you have a baby, but after six months, there are lots of ways to get exercising — the best is to start walking and move up from there. She added in an extra walk five days of the week with the baby, that's approximately three hours of extra exercise. I also suggested she start back at the gym slowly and go one weekend day when she is able to get out without the kids; that's another hour into the right side of her scales.

Feedback after one week of changes

"I found it hard for the first couple of days not to look for something sweet for breakfast or morning tea, but after day three it clicked that I wasn't having sweets until the kids came home from school. I needed that little push to get back into exercising; I loved the morning walks and am enjoying getting back into the gym. I don't think I realised what bad habits I had got into with my sweet snacking until it was pointed out to me, and I was ready to break those habits."

Tips for Sweet Losers

1. Hold off sweet eating until after a certain time (maybe 3 p.m.). If you start with something sweet for breakfast, it initiates the sugar cravings, and then you need to feed them all day. That means no jam or honey on toast, sweet cereal or sugar on cereal, or even flavoured yoghurts. Aim for high-fibre, healthy cereal or eggs.

Make morning tea a savoury snack of dry biscuits or a piece of fresh fruit.

2.Buy your second-favourite type of chocolate. If you buy your favourite, you won't be able to stop at one piece — you'll eat it until it's gone. So buy one you like, but don't have to gorge on all day. The same applies to sweet biscuits or cakes: Go for second or third favourite.

3.Curb your baking. You may love it and it's great for the family, but cut your sweet baking just while you're trying to lose weight on Lazy Loser. Get inventive with healthy recipes.

4.Count out the sweet treats. Don't eat them straight from the pack or off the block; put the amount you're going to eat on a plate, seal the box or block, and put it way out of sight.

5.Get someone to hide your treats. If you live with someone, ask them to help you out by putting your sweet cravings in a place you'll never find them.

Super Loser

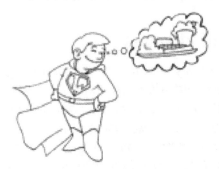

These Losers are the hardest to pin down. More than likely, they're mystified as to why they're overweight or having trouble with their weight. As I've said, the first question I ask Lazy Loser clients is, "What is the main reason you're overweight or struggling to lose weight?" More often than not, Super Loser can't give me an answer.

I'm usually told, "I eat really healthy. I hardly ever have takeaway food, don't binge on sugary snacks, only drink occasionally, and eat five veggies and two fruits daily." According to them, they should be lean, mean, healthy machines, but yet here they are standing in front of me, fat (or fattish). How can it be — are they just freaks of nature, or science gone mad? I try to get to the bottom of it.

Sample day plan of a Super Loser

Pre-breakfast: Glass of juice.

Breakfast: Bowl of untoasted muesli, low-fat milk, piece of toast with margarine and Vegemite.

Morning tea: Low-fat muffin bar, flat white.

Lunch: Two rounds of toasted ham-and-cheese sandwiches on wholemeal with black coffee.

Afternoon tea: Muesli bar.

Dinner: Grilled steak and veggies: Potatoes, corn, peas, and broccoli.

Dessert: Bowl of homemade stewed apples and custard.

Other daily fluid intake: Four glasses of water and two cups of green tea.

For energy output, Super Loser walked the dog very briskly for half an hour after dinner.

Looking at his eating plan, Super Loser seems to be right: It's a mystery. After seeing a balanced diet of meat, fruit, veggies, and whole grains, I had to do more digging.

Me: "Is this just a one-off, or the usual food plan?"

Super Loser: "This is very normal for me. I don't experiment much with food, and unless I go out, which is rare, this is my normal routine."

Me: "Tell me the serving sizes of the foods you eat, or if you don't know, show me the general size with your hands (luckily, we were in a café and there were plates, bowls, and cups for comparing)."

A-ha! The response to this question solved the problem.

Americans have the biggest sweet tooth in the world: They consume an average of 69 kg of sweet based foods per person annually, while Australians take in 47 kg per person.

Let's start with the OJ. I had a normal-sized water glass in front of me (about 250 ml). Super Loser said his orange-juice glass was twice that size, and filled to the top. Therefore, Super Loser starts the day with two glasses of orange juice.

I showed Super Loser a normal bowl, and he revealed the bowls at home were much larger. They're more like pasta bowls, which Super Loser pours food into halfway. In my estimation, he had three servings of muesli. Now we're on a roll.

The toasted sandwiches had two slices of ham and cheese in each (that's four slices each, along with the four slices of bread). There was butter inside the sandwiches and on the outer sides to toast them, as well as a good dollop of homemade chutney on each.

I was taking notes on an A3 piece of paper, I gave it to Super Loser and asked him to fold it into the size of his steak. He folded it in half! That's a big hunk of meat. He insisted it was a good cut with not an ounce of fat on it; however, it was still three servings of steak. Then we got to the two potatoes. There was a bowl of fruit on the counter, and Super Loser said each potato was about the size of a Granny Smith apple. He also had a full corn cob, about a cup of peas, and a big hunk of broccoli.

One thing left: The stewed apples and custard. It was in the same bowl size as the breakfast one, and half full. That could easily be four apples stewed down with 8 tsp. of sugar and a cup of custard.

Any wonder I tag this one Super Loser — that dinner is a lot of food in one sitting. And then off for a half-hour walk with the dog, I've had to run marathons to get rid of meals like that.

These are not Super servings — they're Super-Duper servings. I feel sorry for Super Losers, as often they have no idea the mistakes they're making. The food looks healthy, it's fresh, they're abstaining from packaged goods and drinks, so surely they're doing the right thing . . . but I'm afraid that's not the case. Think of the Lazy Loser scales: The energy-in side is overloaded — no matter what's on there, it's still too much and will make you fat, especially if the energy output side has so little on it. This Super Loser is a truck driver: He sits all day at work, and the half hour dog walk is not making a dent in his output scales.

Often, Super Losers are products of parents who fed them up big with lots of healthy, fresh foods on plates (and seconds if they wanted). These children may have been sporty and active and could burn food as quickly as they could look at it. Then we get to adulthood and are buying our own food and preparing it, and we do what we know. Cook lots, throw it all on an overflowing plate, and eat the lot, not daring to waste a morsel. Super Losers think that's a normal serving size; it's the only amount they know.

Tell-tale signs of a Super Loser?

• You have always been a big eater

• You very rarely feel full

• When you eat or drink your plate, bowl and cup is filled to the brim

• You often have seconds

• At all you can eat buffets you go back and fill your plate more than once

• You eat more than one course at dinner

• You never order a small serve of any type of food

• You think upsized meals are normal servings

Super's tweaks

So what do I do with poor misguided Super Loser — cut him back to normal, standard serving sizes?

Are you kidding? He would starve to death — or at least, that's the way the way he'd feel. If I cut back all Super Loser's food to standard sizes, that would be less than half of what he eats now. It would be like a strict diet to him, and he'd be hungry and turn to snack foods to fill him up.

As I've said, PDB (Poor Dumb Body) gets used to things; Super Loser is happy and comfortable with the food above, halving it will cause chaos. What he needs to do is start cutting some back, so the body hardly notices and the input scales get a bit lighter.

New Super Loser eating plan

Pre-breakfast: Half a glass of juice. Not enough? Fill the glass to the top with water.

Breakfast: Once again, choices are best, it's in Super Loser's control:

• Option 1: Have half the serving of muesli and milk (it may help to buy smaller bowls), and one piece of toast with a scrape of butter and vegemite.

• Option 2: Have the big bowl of muesli and milk, but skip the toast.

Morning tea: Medium banana and flat white made with skim milk.

Lunch: Give the toasted sandwiches a break: Make a fresh salad sandwich. Choose one slice of ham or one slice of cheese — not both — and top it up with salad, like tomatoes, onion, beetroot, and lettuce. Use, butter, mayo, or chutney . . . only one spread (your choice).

Afternoon tea: Piece of fresh fruit.

Dinner: Grilled steak and veggies: Potatoes, corn, peas, and broccoli. Take a quarter off what used to be on your dinner plate. That's a quarter off the steak, one big potato cut in half (it will feel like two), and a quarter off the rest of the veggies.

Dessert: Bowl of homemade stewed apples and low-fat custard, but once again, get a smaller bowl and halve this — that's half the stewed apple and half the custard (make the custard with skim milk).

For energy output, walk the dog very briskly for 45 minutes after dinner. That's only an extra 15 minutes; you and the dog will hardly notice. Do at least an hour a day of other exercise on the days off work.

How much fruit and vegetables should you eat daily? Australia says five vegetables and pieces of fruit, the Brits recommend seven veggies and two fruits, the French are told to eat 10 vegetable portions a day, the Canadians between five and 10, and the Japanese 13 vegetables and four pieces of fruit.

Results on Super's Lazy Loser scales

Left side: Food and drink

• The major change was cutting bits off each serving size. Breakfast was still large and Super Loser had a couple of choices, but the amount eaten was about one quarter less than usual. Dinner had a quarter off all of what he normally ate.

• Stopping the toasting of the sandwiches is good: It removes some butter and cheese. Salad sandwiches are more filling, and Super Loser likes to feel full.

• Adding in fresh fruit for snacks instead of the packaged bars.

• Reducing all dairy to low-fat and skim (e.g. milk in coffee and custard).

It still seems like a lot of food, and it is, but I stripped a quarter off the intake. There is plenty to eat and to keep Super Loser from feeling like he's starving. I haven't changed any of the food choices, so PDB (Poor Dumb Body) won't complain too much.

Right side: Output

Super Loser isn't doing enough to burn all that food off. His job doesn't help, but adding 15 to 30 minutes onto the dog walk and devoting an hour to exercise on each day off work is a start. That's an extra five hours of activity a week.

The first thing I ask Super Losers when they've completed their first week is, "Were you hungry over the week?" More often than not, they say, "No not at all", and that response tells me a lot. They soon realise they were eating to excess because that's what they thought was normal. Taking a bit away wasn't enough to make them hungry, as there was too much there in the first place.

If this system is working well — weight isn't piling on or they're losing weight slowly — I suggest Super Losers stick with this plan for a month. Let the body adapt and get used to the smaller servings.Then when things stabilise and more weight loss is wanted, we attack again by getting the servings back to a normal, standard size. Not on all meals — start with breakfast, get used to that idea, monitor the hunger, then move on to lunch, etc. And of course, there's always plenty of opportunity to add to the energy scales. Another 15 minutes a day won't hurt Super Loser or SD (Super Dog)!

Feedback after one week of changes

"I had no idea how much food I had been eating and the large serving sizes. Breakfast was easy; the fresh salad sandwiches at lunch were more filling than the toasted variety; I missed my large steaks a bit, but I found getting out for the brisk walk straight after dinner soon made me forget the hunger and when I got back, I was fine and not hungry at all."

Tips for Super Losers

1. Buy new crockery! Keep your dinner plate, as you need to see the edges; this is normal. However, some bowls and glasses are too big. Normal-sized cereal bowls and low-ball glasses are best to curb large servings.

2. Check the serving sizes on packets. If something says its two servings, then you need to eat half, not all of it.

3. It may be easier to buy some kitchen scales until you get used to the correct serving sizes of foods. Once you know, you'll find it easy to serve up the right sizes for yourself, but it could take a few weeks.

4. Take a quarter off your dinner plate. If you only change one thing, this is the best one. That means a quarter off everything: Meat, veggies, rice, pasta, all of it. You don't have to waste food — maybe you could cook less, or give the extra to another person in your family or the dog.

5. Drinks have serving sizes as well, so supersized coffees that come in bowls now are like having two coffees. Go back to small coffees, juices, and drinks. If you like a big juice, pour 250 ml into a glass and fill the rest with ice or water.

Fruits and vegetables are not just good for physical health. Studies show people who eat seven to eight portions a day feel more cheerful, loved, and optimistic about the future.

Piggy Loser

Can you guess what problems Piggy Loser has with food and drink?

Sample day plan of a Piggy Loser

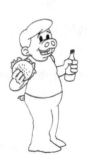

Breakfast: Small tub of low-fat yoghurt.

Morning tea: Banana.

Lunch: 10 dry biscuits with a tomato salsa dip.

Afternoon tea: Cappuccino.

Dinner: Grilled chicken and five servings of steamed vegetables.

Dessert: Nil

Exercise is also formally nil, but he works in construction and is on his feet working hard all day; once, he used a pedometer, and found he walked over 11,000 steps in an eight-hour shift.

What could I possibly say about this day of eating? If anything, there's not enough food in there, but Piggy Loser insists he was not hungry during the day.

Still can't figure out what Piggy Loser's problem is?

I had a bit of trouble getting my head around looking at this Lazy Loser who was at least 30 kg overweight and correlating the food he'd consumed, so of course I needed more information.

Soon all was revealed: This was a Monday food plan, coming off what Piggy Loser said was a horrendous weekend of pigging out! I asked Piggy Loser to write up the weekend for me. He wasn't keen, couldn't remember most of it, and didn't want to remember the other bit. Of course I insisted, so this is what I got:

Saturday

Breakfast/morning tea: Nothing — slept in.

Lunch: McDonalds upsized meal deal: Burger, large fries, large coke, and a sundae. Said this was his junk-food treat for the week.

Afternoon tea: Four stubbies of regular beer and bags of chips, nuts, cheese, and biscuits shared with friends (no idea how much food, but lots).

Dinner: Huge chicken schnitzel with gravy, hot chips, all-you-can-eat salad bar, small plate of coleslaw, potato salad, two pieces of garlic bread, and two pots of beer at a pub.

Night out at pubs/clubs: He lost count, but at least 10 rum and cokes over six hours.

Late-night snack: Lamb kebab and one slice of pizza out of a friend's box.

Sunday

Breakfast/morning tea/lunch: He felt pretty hung over, so nothing.

Afternoon: Spent time at a friend's watching footy on TV and had six stubbies of regular beer and lots of snack foods over four hours. He grabbed a takeaway medium pizza on the way home, and washed it down with Coke.

Mystery solved! When Piggy Loser goes off the rails, it's right into an eating-and-drinking ditch. Usually it's on the weekend, but binges have been known to happen on weekdays as well. In most of Piggy Loser's weeks, he goes from feeling guilty, sick or hung over on Monday from all that rubbish to hungry and deprived by Friday. But by the weekend, Piggy Loser is on the attack and loses all control.

It's not a nice or healthy way to live: Piggy Loser is either feeling guilty, hungry, and deprived, or stuffed with so much food and drink he feels sick.

Tell-tale signs of a Sweet Loser?

- You can never stop at one of anything
- Once a packet of food is open its gone- in your belly
- You have a food or drink splurge at least once a week
- You feel guilty after the splurging
- You are always trying to be good!
- You often feel sick after a food splurge
- Sometimes you can splurge all day or for several days

Piggy's tweaks

There's really only one thing to do: Break the pig-out cycle and stop the starvation and guilt. It's a roller coaster over the week — the pigging out is causing the weight gain and counteracts the healthy minimal eating during the week. Piggy Loser doesn't only need to change the way he eats, but also needs to change his attitude towards the way he eats, which is hard.

Like Tipsy Loser, all alcohol should be halved. Piggy eats out a lot on weekends; that's okay, but he needs to choose healthier options off the menu and not overeat.

One thing Piggy Loser can do to help curb the pig-out is put lots of physical activity into the weekend. That way, the food and drink at least has a chance to be burned off before Monday comes around.

New Piggy Loser eating plan

Breakfast: Low-fat yoghurt and a bowl of healthy cereal or two pieces of toast (yoghurt is not enough).

Morning tea: Banana.

Lunch: 10 small dry biscuits with tomato salsa dip and a piece of fruit.

Afternoon tea: Cappuccino with skim milk and an apple.

Dinner: Grilled chicken and five servings of steamed vegetables.

Dessert: Fruit or low-fat ice cream.

Australians over the age of 15 drink an average of 10.4 litres of alcohol a year per person. However, that is not our highest figure; the peak was recorded way back in the 1830s, when we drank 13.6 litres per person 15+. It halved to under 6 litres per person in the 1890s due to an economic downturn; the Great Depression saw it half again to only 2.9 litres per head. After WWII, it rose slowly until another high peak in 1975, hitting 13.1 litres per person. It has decreased slowly to the round 10.4 litres today; broken down, it works out as 4.23 litres of beer, 3.74 of wine, 1.32 of spirits, and .7 of pre mixed drinks.

That bit's easy. Now for weekend Piggy Loser . . .

Saturday

Breakfast: This shouldn't be missed! Try poached eggs on toast to set you up for the day.

Morning tea: Banana.

Lunch: Bowl of salad with feta cheese.

Now for the drinking. Like Tipsy Loser, all alcohol should be halved—try two light strength beers (once you get drunk, all control goes out the window). If snacks come out, have your own bowl, count out 20 chips or nuts, and eat slowly. That's it for snack food.

Dinner: Everyone off to the pub. All breaded meat is off limits — so no more schnitzels! Order grilled chicken or steak; if having chips, eat 10 only and give the rest to someone else (or, if you can't do that, ask for no chips). At the salad bar, don't have white salads — they have lots of creamy dressings. Get a green salad, beetroot, or tabbouli salad, or just tomato, lettuce, etc. Give the garlic bread a miss — it's not needed.

Party time: Once again, halve the drinks; five rums made with diet soft drink. Don't go in rounds with your friends; or have a drink every second round instead. Drink water in between each rum. You're still drinking all night (with hopefully half the hangover).

After party: You know you don't need the kebab, but if you can't resist, share one with your friend (get it cut in half).

Sunday

Okay, the big weekend of pigging out ends now. You've had great time with plenty to eat and drink, but it has to get back on track today— back to a normal healthy eating plan, just like on weekdays.

I know the above plan still looks like a pig-out, but it's really half a pig-out, and that's better than a full-on one. There are lots of rewards in there, and no social dilemmas of not being able to go out and have fun with friends because you can't eat or drink.

This is the start of downscaling the pig-out. Once the half pig-out gets accepted, it will start to feel like a full one, so that will then get scaled back to half of that pig-out, and so on. The few extra weekday snacks will keep hunger at bay and not make Piggy

Loser crave for the weekend to come so he can wallow in rubbishy foods the whole time. In Piggy Loser's case, he takes some of the weekend pig-out and puts it into the starving days to balance the whole week — not just the scales.

For energy out, walking lots at work is great and helps, but often the Piggy Loser suffers mentally with his eating — and we all know exercise helps keep us upbeat and happier. Piggy Loser needs to exercise, especially on weekends when he has the time to do more than just eat and drink.

Piggy was given four exercise rules to follow over the weekend:

1. Saturday morning: Get up and walk, run, or go to gym. This starts the day right, and gets the endorphins kicked in for the weekend.

2. After the afternoon splurge and before the huge night out, another 45 minutes of exercise has to be added in. A good one is to leave the car at home and walk to the pub.

3. Sunday morning: Hung over and can't face food? Drink water, and before anything else, do a one-hour walk or run. The best thing for a hangover is exercise, as it gets rid of all that alcohol and you will feel better afterwards. By the time you get back, the urge for the hair of the dog may be gone!

4. Sunday afternoon: Replace the afternoon drinking session with a sporty session. Get your mates together for a few hours of social cricket, a footy match, a tennis game or a bush walk or run. You get the social connection, and lots of energy goes out — not in.

Even if Piggy Loser doesn't exercise during the week, these four sessions stuck bang in the middle of peak-hour pigging out will break the mental cycle and get rid of some of the extra calories.

Another good reason to slot plenty of activity in is even if Saturday night's drinking and splurging goes out of control (which, let's face it, can happen), at least by Sunday evening the guilt fest will not be crippling Piggy Loser into starvation mode on Monday, as he will tell himself, "Well, at least I exercised plenty."

> Overeating, poor memory formation, learning disorders, and depression have all been linked in recent research to the over-consumption of sugar.

Results on Piggy's Lazy Loser scales

Left side: Food and drink

• The major change was cutting the two-day pig-out to one. That's half off the input.

• The Saturday pig-out was halved as well, with half the drinks and snacks and a healthier pub dinner.

Right side: Output

Piggy Loser was spending lots of time with his friends on weekends, but mostly it was spent sitting, eating, and drinking. Changing one of those sessions to an active one meant they were still together having fun, but Piggy Loser could burn off energy as well. Also, Piggy Loser's weekdays became more active due to him not carrying guilt over Sunday's pig-out.

Feedback after one week of changes

"I thought cutting back to one pig-out (or drinking session) a week would be hard, but it turned out to be a lot easier than I thought. I told a few mates that I wasn't drinking on Sunday and asked who was up for a few hours of tennis, and four were really keen. We had a great time and are going to do this every Sunday. I didn't feel so fat and guilty on Monday, and I found I had more energy: I wasn't hung over for the first three days of the week, so I could exercise on those days."

Tips for Piggy Loser

1. Pig-outs should not last all day and night; nominate one pig-out a week and stick with it. Maybe its Saturday night when you go out with friends or Sunday afternoon when you have a few beers and watch the footy, but it can't be both. Decide before the weekend comes around when you're going to have your pig-out, and that's it.

2. Nominate yourself as the designated driver, and have a drink-free night. You can still dance and have fun — just don't pig out.

3. Pig out on exercise. You have lots of friends to go out and drink with, so get those same friends to exercise with you. Each weekend,

organise a game of social footy, or doubles round-robin tennis or cricket; go for a big bush walk or a run. Get outside for hours, and you'll burn all the pig-out calories while still hanging with the people you enjoy being around the most.

4. Don't open packets of food! Piggy Losers usually can't stop at one of anything —once the pack is open, it's gone. Make that one of your rules: You'll never open a packet of food. If it's already open, you may gorge the lot, but at least it hopefully wasn't a full packet. If you live on your own and have to open a package of food, buy small, individual snacks instead of big packs.

Lazy Bottom Line

• Everyone has their own temptations and weaknesses when it comes to food and exercise. Finding out what yours are, why you do them, and starting to tweak them is the first step to stop gaining weight.

• The above outlines are only general, and you may see bits of yourself in all of them. It's best to focus on the major thing that is stopping you from losing weight or getting healthy, and work on that first. Once you get that sorted, look at some of the other categories and see what can be tweaked there.

• I've mentioned in other chapters that drinks are one of the major causes of overweight people not being able to lose weight, and they should be avoided —even the zero-calorie ones — yet here I am recommending low-calorie mixers for alcohol. This is to help tweak the extra calories that come when alcohol is in the diet: Low-calorie mixers take out some of the energy in, but overall it's still an alcoholic drink. Consuming soft drinks on a daily basis as a replacement for water is adding in sugar and sugar cravings; that is part of Sweet Loser's problem, it should start off halved or cut out of his or her daily plan.

• On any of the plans, the main idea is to take out something from the input side and add more energy to the output side. The above examples are hints and tips on how that can be done, but you need to write up your own plan and alter it to get the balance right for you.

• Don't fall into the trap of cutting back your temptations on the left-hand side to zero — this would mean no alcohol for Tipsy; zero in-between snacks for Moo; no chocolate or cake for Sweet; going back to minimum serving sizes for Super: and no going out on weekends for Piggy — and thinking this will speed up weight loss. It may in the short term, but your cravings will start to kick in and it won't take long for you to be back at the start. Begin with baby steps. If you want to speed things up, add activity to the right side; this formula will be more successful.

Be grateful you live on earth: If you lived on Jupiter, you'd weigh two and half times what you do now!

Lazy Loser

Chapter 18 – Lazy Loser Best Tips

Most of the following topics have been discussed in the previous 17 chapters, but I think they bear repeating. This chapter is full of the tips and tricks that I live by. Even if you only do two or three of these things, you'll exert some control over your eating and general health, so give it a go.

Don't buy your favourites

Say you're a chocoholic (as I've said, there is no such thing, but it's such a great label), and your favourite is Turkish delight (guess who likes Turkish delight?) . . . so don't buy Turkish delight! If I buy Turkish delight chocolate, there's no telling what will happen. Well there is, actually: I'll eat it all! I'm like the poor Vikings being lured by the naughty mermaids; it calls out to me from the fridge or pantry, and won't let me be until it's in my belly!

Therefore, I rarely buy delicious Turkish delight. I still buy and eat chocolate — just not my favourite. Chocolate with macadamia nuts talks to me as well, I try to avoid it as well. Now, you could say just don't buy chocolate . . . but are you crazy? Life without chocolate is a life I don't want to be involved in.

There are many types of chocolate I like, can eat, and don't go silly over. I often buy a small block of dairy-milk plain chocolate and find two small pieces satisfy me without the need to devour the lot. My third-favourite chocolate doesn't have the same talking capacity and control over me that Turkish delight and nutty chocolate have.

Do the same thing yourself when it comes to your very favourite food fetish. Do you love blue cheese that you can't stop eating it until the whole chunk has gone? You can still have your gourmet cheese — but buy your second- or third-favourite type.

Would you sell your kids for chocolate-chip ice cream? Buy a flavour you like, but can stop at one or two scoops with. When you're standing in your favourite aisle of the supermarket and being pulled like a magnet to your yummiest thing, STOP. Move a little to the left or right and get the second- or third-yummiest thing; it will still taste great and you'll enjoy it, but you won't devour it all in one sitting.

Does that mean you never get to eat your favourite foods? No! Treat yourself on special occasions, or drop hints for birthdays and Christmas.

Serving sizes

The discrepancy in the food industry of recommended serving sizes is disgraceful. If you are overweight or a big eater and want to cheat the system, just walk along the aisle and find the brand that has the largest serving sizes, and that's the one for you. But in reality, you're only cheating yourself in the end.

It's not the national food authority that states the serving sizes of foods — it's the manufacturers, and they have the power to list whatever they want.

A survey by the food standards committee in Australia found discrepancies in most packaged foods, with some serving sizes being three or more times that of an exact same product of a different brand. They even found the same companies had different serving sizes on their own brands.

You are what you eat — so don't be fake, easy, fast, or cheap!

Confusion is rife for the food consumer, so the best way is to take charge yourself. Read Chapter 10: Don't Count or Read . . . Just Look. It gives my Lazy rundown of what you should be eating in a day, from food groups to how to estimate serving size. Once you know what size steak you should eat in one sitting; how much cereal to pour into your bowl; what the amount of rice should look like on your plate, etc., you'll be set for life. I suggest you disregard the suggested or recommended serving sizes on food packets and go with your own.

Stop the overflow

This follows on from serving sizes. If you can't see the rim or your dinner plate, or the food is within 2.5 cm (1") of the edge, there's too much on your plate. If your cereal bowl or soup or salad bowl is filled to the very top, it's too much. Leave a 2.5 cm (1") rim around your plates and bowls when you put your food into them. If you can't see your dining companions over the high mound of food on your plate, it's time to prune! The mound should be no higher than 3 cm (1.2"). Don't dine with a ruler handy? Try three finger widths.

And don't go buying smaller crockery to make it look like you're eating more, or to try and trick your mind into seeing a big pile of food on a small plate. You're not a child, and shouldn't have to dine like one. If you know how your normal dinner plate should look and how much space is left in your bowl, that's a good thing.

Don't eat randomly!

Never eat straight from the packet. Put the food you're about to consume in a bowl or on a plate, where you can see exactly how much you'll be eating. Eating biscuits, chips, nuts, lollies, or even so-called healthy snacks directly from a packet means you have no idea how much you're eating — or you know when the packet is empty, and by then it's too late.

> The average woman spends 31 years of her life trying to lose weight.

Count your snacks

Another take on the above is to count all the snacks you dish up for yourself. Set a limit: 20 is a good number, or 30 for tiny snacks and five to 10 for larger nibblies. Look at the size of the snack and make a decision. Count out 30 sultanas, peanuts, or dried cranberries; for larger snacks: 20 potato chips, pecans or macadamias, rice crackers, grapes, or blueberries. For larger snacks: five dried apricots or strawberries. Once you've counted out your snack, seal the remaining packet and put it back where it came from: The pantry.

Food science gone mad

The continual carry on about food science in the 21st century is confusing and frustrating. Food science is giving food too much power — power it doesn't even want. It's also giving food manufacturers license to play with scientific results to purport claims about their products to try and impress the ignorant consumer.

I was never good at science, because it never looked appealing. I'm good at food, as to me, it looks very appealing! We can't see calories, nutrients, enzymes, preservatives, or food additives when we look at our food; why don't we just deal with what we can see?

Look at your dinner plate. Does it have a serving of lean meat and a colourful array of vegetables on it? There you go — thumbs up. Does it have protein, vitamins and minerals, no food preservatives or food additives? That's a double thumbs up. How many calories does it have? Who knows, but if it covers all the other bases, it must be good.

Take back your power and confidence when it comes to feeding you and your family. If you're eating fresh vegetables and fruits, lean meat (fish or chicken), some dairy and eggs, and unsalted nuts, using olive oil for cooking, curbing your unhealthy snacks, cutting back on packaged and high-sugar food and drink, and preparing your own meals most of the time — that's all the science you need.

And remember, if you're eating too much of one food source, you don't need Einstein to tell you that you may not be having enough of another. As boring as it sounds, "Everything in moderation" — even the stuff scientists give the thumbs-up to.

Stocktake at the end of each day

If you're trying to lose weight and have been off and on for a long time, you probably spend half your time cutting back on calories and eating healthily and the other half off the leash, eating whatever and whenever you want.

All the amount of dieting and healthy eating will never counteract the splurges you have when you're not watching what you are eating. There is nothing wrong with a splurge — we all have them — however, if you're splurging daily for weeks, the kilos pile on, and then it's back to the harsh dieting. You need to stop this yo-yo living.

At the end of each day, I assess what I've eaten. I don't write it down; I do a quick checklist in my head. If there was a chocolate splurge in there, I don't beat myself up about it. I say "Okay, no chocolate tomorrow, back to fruit snacks", or I set the alarm to start the next day with a long run.

At the end of the day, I check in with myself. Here are some of the things I may say:

• "How many veggies did I eat today?" If the answer is none, I say, "Okay, I'll have a big veggie stir-fry tomorrow for dinner, and maybe my homemade veggie soup for lunch."

• "How much did wine did I have today?" I had one glass at lunch with a friend and two glasses at dinner, so two AFDs (Alcohol-Free Days) are coming up.

• "Why was I so hungry today?" I was rushed this morning and skipped brekkie, which made me want food all day. Tomorrow, I'll start the day with two eggs on toast.

> More than 50 years of research confirms that diets have a failure rate of between 95 and 98%. For every 100 people who diet, 98 of them will either lose no weight or will soon regain any weight they do lose.

If you check in with yourself each day, it's easy to see what you did wrong (if anything) and then make amends in the next 24 hours. If you're eating randomly for a month, it's hard to reel it in, as you've already created bad habits and are probably carrying around an extra couple of kilos as well.

This is a simple trick, easy to do, and will become a habit after a while.

Lazy Tale

I married at 21 and had my first child at 22; by 30, I had four darlings, and by 40, I was cooking for four adults and two children.

I'm telling this story to impress upon you that I've spent my adult life cooking for other people (mostly a herd of people). Budget constraints and the health of my family were the prime motivation for me to provide home-cooked, healthy meals. It was easy to buy a huge weekly shop of fresh food (and a few snacks) at the supermarket and green grocer and cook all the meals myself. I didn't need to do a stocktake at the end of each day, as the majority of the food I ate was nutritious and healthy; often, I gnawed on the carcass left after the herd had moved through, and sometimes the pickings were slim!

Things changed in my 50's: Family life got down to one teenager and me. I was still cooking up healthy meals, only to get calls from her saying she was working after school or having dinner with a friend. So there I was, sitting in front of a family dinner for one. Then I'd get lazy and think, *If she isn't going to be home for meals, it's hardly worth cooking. It's easier and cheaper to get takeaway.*

Then I moved out of the home! I was off on my "Lazy Runner" book tour, just me and the road and hotels or B&Bs for four months. For the first time in my life, I wasn't chief cook and bottle washer — I was living like a teenage backpacker. Cooking was often not an option, and my budget didn't allow for restaurant eating.

For the first week, it was a snack fest. I ate bits and pieces all day, with no set meals or eating routine. I would go to the supermarket and fill a bag with things that didn't require any preparation.

On the one hand, it was good: I had no alcohol (I'm not a fan of drinking alone) and I ate lots of fruit because it's perfectly packaged and doesn't require crockery or cutlery! But after a week or two, I didn't feel so bright. I wasn't eating enough meat or vegetables, and was snacking on too many processed foods and drinking way too much coffee.

One night, I did a stocktake . . . and the results were bad. I couldn't remember the last time I'd eaten more than one vegetable in a day or eaten meat, fish, or an egg! I had to set up a new eating plan, or I wouldn't survive the tour. It wasn't easy at first, but after some thought, I soon realised I could eat healthy on the road. But I had to plan better.

I started the day with breakfast out. Eating out at dinner was too expensive, but you can get a good cooked brekkie (eggs on toast) at a reasonable price — and it comes with a coffee! For lunch, I'd buy a fresh wholemeal roll at a bakery and fill it with the single-serving salad bowl many supermarkets have these days; very filling, with lots of vegies. By dinner (with no cooking facilities), I'd be happy to have yoghurt and fruit or nuts, or biscuits and cheese.

I also changed my exercise routine. I've always been a morning runner, but I became an evening exerciser on the tour. Coming from a non-daylight-savings state, I enjoyed being able to run or walk after dinner, and as I didn't have any entertainment (people or TV) and wasn't eating a huge dinner or drinking, I found getting out and exercising at dusk the best thing for me.

In those four months, I upended every food, drink, and exercise pattern I'd built over the last 50 years. I ate well and often, but when I got home, a few people commented that I'd lost weight. I got on the scales and found I'd dropped 3 kg!

It wasn't from dieting or deliberately cutting back any foods or exercising more: It was from changing the way I did things. My main meal was breakfast, and my smallest was dinner. I exercised every evening because I was bored! I hardly drank alcohol, and I reduced my red-meat intake drastically, since I had no way of cooking it and am not a fan of steak tartare! For extra protein, I ate two eggs a day and snacked on nuts. If I hadn't done a stocktake a week into my tour, I would've come back broke and 10 kg heavier.

The moral of this Lazy Tale is that when situations change in your life, you need to change as well. If someone moves out of your home and you continue to cook like that person is still there, the food has to go somewhere — and usually that place is in you. If your job changes and you can't get to the gym as often as you'd like, you have to find some new fitness activity to do.

Often, weight gain comes from years of not adapting to changes in our lives; for example, running after small children and eating lots may have kept you at a steady weight once, but the kids grow up and you are still eating the same amount. As the Lazy Loser scales show, you'll put on weight. A job change from active to sedentary or where you once walked to work but now have to drive as its further away is also a change that will affect your weight if your diet stays the same.

This is why we need to stocktake our food intake regularly (daily or weekly). If you see something out of whack on the left hand side of your scales, you need to make changes to the right hand side as well to get the balance back. Make sure you do it as soon as changes occur, because as time goes by, habits set in and weight goes up.

The dreaded drink

The biggest growth in the food industry is not food: It's flavoured drinks. When I was growing up, I don't remember my mother buying me a drink. "Find a tap" or "You should've had one at home before we left" were the standard replies if I was thirsty. Now, service stations and supermarkets have drink fridges covering one or two walls.

If you're overweight and you drink anything other than water, herbal tea, or a couple of coffees a day, try this: Do nothing else in your diet except stop drinking all other drinks. Just sit back and see what happens.

Two things will happen: Your craving for sugar will decrease, and I bet you'll lose weight (no, not kilos a week but over time). This is for two reasons: The high sugar in the drinks makes you thirstier, so you drink more. The more sugar you have, the more your body craves it, so you look for sugary snacks to wash down your flavoured drinks with.

Don't be fooled by the healthy-looking drinks in the fridges. They may have fruity names and lovely pictures of fresh fruits and veggies on the front, but you're still drinking a large percentage of sugar. They may tell you it's natural sugar or 100% fruit juice, but that natural sugar will still make you fat. Flavoured milks are high in sugar; even if they say "low-fat", they still have the sugar hit of the flavour.

Here are some average sugar amounts for some more popular flavoured drinks:

• Sports drinks: 39 g (equivalent to 10 tsp. sugar)

• Soft drinks and lemonades: 39 g (equivalent to 10 tsp. sugar)

• Vitamin or flavoured waters: 20 to 25 g (equivalent to five to six tsp. sugar)

• A glass of fruit juice: 22 to 30 g (equivalent to six to eight tsp. sugar)

There are approximately 4 g of sugar in a cube of sugar or a teaspoon of sugar; if the figure on your label says 40, that's 10 tsp.

It's recommended that we eat five servings of vegetables and two servings of fruit a day. Only 10% of modern societies attain this level.

As an experiment, try mixing 10 tsp. of white sugar with 375 ml water, and drink it down. I bet it tastes disgusting. But that much sugar in a fizzy drink tastes great, so how can that be? They add flavours and chemicals to make all the sugar taste good!

When you feel like a drink, it's because you're thirsty, not hungry, so think hydration. Water is the best for hydration.

Cut packaged food in half

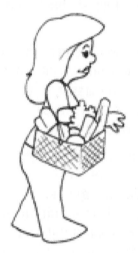

When you get to the register on your next grocery trip, look in your basket or trolley and do a quick estimate. How much is packaged food? How much is unpackaged? If more than half is packaged, then get rid of it — yes, take it out and put it back, or ask the poor cashier to take it back, as you don't want it.

I've been following this rule for years. I actually separate the packaged from the unpackaged in the trolley or basket, and if the "P" section (that's what I call the packaged goods) is bigger than the "UP" section, it has to be cut; no ifs, ands, or buts, I go through the "P"s and decide which is not coming home with me.

Packaged-food products have had a huge growth over the past 20 years. They're everywhere — in fact, 80% of the food in supermarkets is packaged. What I mean by packaged is that it has been processed in some way to get into the packet. It's either cooked or preserved or has had other things added in, like flavourings, colourings, extra sugars or oils, and the odd chemical or two.

Packaged foods are easy to find: They make up all the aisles of the supermarket, and half the outside walls (fridges). It's easier to point out which areas are not processed: The sections outside the aisles (fruits and vegetables, bakery, deli, meat and seafood sections); however, many of the products in these areas are packaged or processed as well.

Now I can hear you hollering at me: "Not all packaged foods are bad and unhealthy!" That's right, but I still like to make sure that half of what I'm eating is fresh and not tampered with.

I'll make allowances, as some of the packaging is a convenient way to get the food out of the supermarket and into your house without ruining it:

• Fresh meat, chicken, or fish in Styrofoam containers and cling wrap are okay. However, if it has had anything else added on the label, then it's processed. This includes things like sausages and all processed meats.

• Real fresh milk in bottles, or yoghurts and cheeses in containers are okay. Finding a cow to milk is a problem, and we need milk products to be pasteurised. However, if the product has more than what came out of an udder, it's processed. A good way to tell is if it's any colour other than white, cream, or yellowish.

• Bread comes in plastic bags. I'll let you decide which is more processed than others.

Packaged foods such as yoghurt, frozen fruits, and frozen vegetables go in the "P" section of your trolley. Remember: You're allowed 50% packaged foods, so make sure you select the right ones. If you're over on two packaged products — for example, the family-sized chips and large tub of yoghurt — you have to choose. Make the right choice for you and your family.

Drink more (water, that is)

You've heard it all before, and no, it doesn't make you skinny unless it's the only thing you consume. However, water can make you feel better. Fatigue, sluggishness, headaches, and even nausea can be caused by not drinking enough water. The feelings I just described can make us flat and grumpy, and then we think we're hungry and reach for some comfort food or drink.

When you think you're hungry, reach for a drink of water first, then wait a few minutes; maybe you were only thirsty.

Between 16,000 and 17,000 new food products turn up in supermarkets annually.

Sit to eat

If I eat while I'm doing something else, I find I don't remember what I ate or what it tasted like. This is bad — especially if what I ate was chocolate (I want to taste that!).

Eating is a no-brainer — you have been doing it all your life, and could do it with your eyes closed. So when you pair it with an activity that requires more thought, like reading, driving, or watching TV, eating will take a backseat.

I love food, and want to enjoy it. If I eat while doing something else and have forgotten what I've eaten, how much, and how good it tasted, I want more. If I sit and eat and taste my food, I feel satisfied and less likely to want to eat again in five minutes.

For these reasons, I don't eat while driving or watching TV. In the past, I've been known to see empty packets of food near me and not be able to figure out who ate them until I accept the sad truth: I did!

Don't skip brekkie

It's my favourite meal of the day, but I know many people don't share my love of breakfast. The first thing in the morning is the only time of the day that hunger is legitimate; at other times in the day, the feeling of hunger is fake, and comes from boredom or the routine of meal breaks we abide by.

When you wake up, you've usually gone for eight to 12 hours without eating; the food you eat at this time is exactly why we eat and need food. It's to get us jump-started and provide nutrients to get us through our busy days. All other meals after this are just little top-ups to keep us going.

You don't have to chow down on a big brekkie of eggs and bacon with all the extras; cereal, toast, fruit, and yoghurt are all good ways to start the day. But once again, don't get sucked into the eat-and-run breakfast bars and drinks: Sit and eat a normal meal (set the alarm 10 minutes earlier, if you need to).

Get rid of those damn scales!

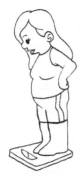

This is a very strong, serious message I have for you, which is why I cursed in the title! I've met many people who are addicted to their bathroom scales. They get on them at least once a day, and sometimes more. And depending on what they see each time they jump on, it dictates their mood for the day and what they eat as well. Don't like what you see? "What the hell, I'm going to have a pig-out." Like what you see? "Yaaayyy, I deserve a special treat!"

Scales can fluctuate between 1 and 3 kg a day, but fat can't go on and come off that quickly. Therefore, it's not a true reading — maybe it's reflecting hydration levels, or your scale is temperamental. Whatever it is, it's going to cause you grief at some point.

If you need to check your weight, do it once a month. Write it in your diary, and do it at the same time of the day each month. My scale-addicted Lazy Losers have nicknamed their scales Elvis, as I tell them the scales must leave the building after a weigh-in! Change your bathroom scales to garage scales — you won't be as tempted to go out and get them with your bath towel wrapped around you.

Eat when you're hungry or want to eat

This one is easier said than done; society has fixed meal routines, and they can be hard to ignore. Family, school, and work all dictate when we should eat, and what type of food we should consume at each sitting. Many people down tools at 12 p.m. to have lunch whether they're hungry or not: Out comes the lunch box, and we eat a meal that is often too large and unneeded.

Since becoming an adult (zillions of years ago), I haven't regularly eaten what society would label lunch (the midday meal). I find I'm

> The Fat Whisperer: Hollywood's (it could only happen there) Mary Ascension Saulnier says she can talk fat cells out of the body. "I listen to what emotion is in the cell membrane," she says. "Then . . . tell the cell which way to move out of the body."

not ready for food yet. I like a good breakfast, so when the usual lunch hour ticks around, I'm not hungry.

It helps that I work my own hours and have the freedom to eat when I want. Often, I'm peckish at 3 or 4 p.m., which is when I usually have a snack of fruit, cheese, or dip and biscuits, and maybe a chocolate something! If you're at work or school, lunch is at 12 or 1 p.m. If you are not hungry, don't have lunch. Yes, I hear you once again, gasping with horror: "How will I get through the day if I don't eat the midday meal? I'll starve!"

If you have to take a lunch break at work, school, or university and you're not hungry, use the break to do something else. Slot in your daily exercise hour, go for a walk, run some errands, or work through lunch if you're busy. Then when you're feeling hungry later at 2, 3, or 4 p.m., have the fruit, yoghurt, or the sandwich you made (you may have to take your food with you, as lunch in our society is usually over by 2 p.m.).

Two positives will come from this: You'll enjoy your food more when you eat at the time you're feeling hungry, and you'll have extra freedom to use your lunch break the way you want.

Eat less

I've mentioned this many times: We eat too much. Serving sizes have grown and often doubled over the past 20 years, and in turn, we're growing. On the occasions I have told my Lazy Losers to take a quarter off the usual amount on their dinner plate and then ask a week later if they went to bed hungry, 95% of the time, the reply is "No" — they were satisfied with the reduced servings. This proves we don't need as much food as we think. As my mother used to say, "Our eyes are too large for our bellies!"

Most of us eat out more these days and tend to eat whatever is dished up to us. Even if it's huge, we try to eat as much as we can without exploding, our parents' voices ringing in our ears — "Eat everything on your plate — think of the poor starving kids in Africa!"

If you don't like the thought of wasting food; don't order as much or share a meal with a friend, or partner. Ask for a half size meal.

Never upsize, no matter how much cheaper it sounds — it will cost you in the long run!

Speak up. If you're serving yourself, that's easier, but if partners or parents are dumping huge portions on your plate, say, "No, that's too much", or "Only half of that, please." You can do it. If portion sizes are an issue for you, steer clear of buffets and other all-you-can-eat restaurants.

Fast food is okay, but not too often

Fast–food outlets are in our faces daily: On most TV ad breaks, on every corner as you drive home, through deals in your letterbox, etc. The general claims made are that it's easier and cheaper than preparing your own meals (not to mention saves cleaning up afterwards), and it appeals to our lazy natures.

If you're a fast-food junkie, you should aim to cut back to one fast meal a week. The problem with fast-food meals is they usually contain more sugar, salt, and fat, and they aren't as nutritionally balanced as the meals you prepare at home.

However, not all fast foods are created equal. Here are you best options:

• Thin-crust pizzas with less meat and cheese. Remember my rule for the salad sandwich: Only meat or cheese, not both. Opt for vegetarian with cheese or one meat, and if you need the cheese, ask for half (you can do it). Chicken is better than oily salami, bacon, and ham varieties.

• Skinless or grilled chicken options for your burgers and wraps.

• Souvlaki or Doner kebabs. These often have lots of veggies with grilled meats. Watch out for the creamy sauces and dressings, though — opt for one sauce, and make it non-creamy.

• Grilled fish or lean-meat hamburgers, freshly made.

• Sushi.

> Two-thirds of food advertising is spent promoting processed foods, soft drinks, and alcohol.

- Asian stir-fries with grilled meat and lots of veggies, served with steamed rice.

- Jacket potatoes served without cream sauces or butter; opt for baked beans, salads, or veggies.

- Salad and sandwich bars. Keep an eye on sandwich fillings — meatballs, crumbed or breaded meats, and salami-type meats can make your sandwich high in fat. Choose lean ham or chicken, leave off the cheese, and choose only one sauce or dressing. Same goes for the healthy-looking bowls of salad: If it's covered in thick, creamy dressing, it won't be as healthy as a green salad.

The biggest mistake we make with fast food is adding on chips, fries, onion rings, hash browns, etc. If you leave those things out of the equation, you'll be cutting out between 30 and 50 g of fat. To lose weight, we should eat less than 40 g of fat, and you've made a big dent in your fat consumption right there. If you have to have fries, follow my rule of 10 only, and then pass them onto someone else to finish off.

Be nice

My final tip and word for Lazy Loser: Be nice to yourself! You're the one you have to live with forever, so stop beating yourself up at every turn in life.

Here are some ways to be nice to yourself:

- Enjoy food — after keeping you alive, enjoyment is the second reason it was invented. It's only food and drink you're consuming, not toxins and poison. Every now and again, savour every morsel of a treat without guilt.

- Have fun. Do things you enjoy for no other reason than to feel good and happy.

- Don't be so hard on PDB (Poor Dumb Body) — it's your best buddy, not the enemy. Give it some direction, but don't keep picking on it; if it wasn't for PDB, you wouldn't be here.

- Be optimistic. Things will change for you if you're confident about the future and have a Lazy Loser plan in place. It doesn't matter when, but it will happen.

• Be thankful. You live in a great world, with wonderful choices in all areas: Healthy food, good drinking water, freedom, a safe environment, and the ability to do or be anything you want.

• Accept yourself. If you don't know who you are or what you want to be, go find out! Life's too short for uncertainty. If you're not happy with you, no one will be happy with you. Change what you can, and accept what you can't.

And be diet-free for the rest of your days.

Lazy Bottom Line

• Don't buy your favourite treats — opt for your second or third best ones. This way you will not devour the lot in one sitting — save your favourites for special occasions.

• Stop eating too much — look at everything you are about to eat and make an assessment, if it's too much, remove a quarter from your bowl or plate.

• If you drink soft drinks, fruit juices, vitamin waters or sports drinks every day — try stopping. Sit back and see what happens to your weight after a month.

• Eat meals when you feel like eating or are hungry — don't get into the trap of eating when you don't feel like it- do something else on meal breaks and eat later when you are hungry.

• Sit and eat breakfast every day; drink more water; only have fast or takeaway food once a week and if you have to weigh yourself do it once a month — no more.

• Monitor your grocery shopping. Look in your trolley or basket before you get to the checkout — if more of your food is packaged or in plastic than fresh unpackaged food, put some back!

• Be Happy and enjoy life.

Food that goes bad in a week or less is good for you.

Lazy Loser